THE COMPLETE GUIDE TO
WEIGHT LOSS

Paul Waters

B L O O M S B U R Y

LONDON · NEW DELHI · NEW YORK · SYDNEY

Published by Bloomsbury Publishing Plc
50 Bedford Square
London WC1B 3DP
www.bloomsbury.com

Bloomsbury is a trademark of Bloomsbury Publishing Plc

First edition 2014
Copyright © 2014 Paul Waters
ISBN (print): 978-1-4729-0317-4
ISBN (ePdf): 978-1-4729-0316-7
ISBN (EPUB): 978-1-4729-0315-0

Acknowledgements
Cover photograph © Shutterstock
Inside photographs © Gerard Brown, with the exception of pages: ix © Zia Soleil / Iconica / Getty Images; x, 6, 13, 75, 77, 91, 103, 119, 129, 155, 157, 158, 160, 164 and 171 © Shutterstock; 114 Geoff Caddick / PA Archive / PA Images; and 177 © Michael Conroy / AP/ PA Images
Illustrations by Perspectiv Design, with the exception of page 101 (left) © Shutterstock; (right) © Crown copyright 2013
Commissioned by Charlotte Croft

Typeset in 10.75pt on 14pt Adobe Caslon by seagulls.net

Printed and bound in China by Toppan Leefung Printing

10 9 8 7 6 5 4 3 2 1

CONTENTS

DEFINITION OF TERMS

Throughout the book the following terms are used consistently:

Weight loss – in this context it refers to any reduction in body weight, although it relates to the loss of fat and not lean tissue. At times it is used interchangeably with 'fat loss'.

Weight maintenance – the maintenance of weight loss/fat loss for a sustained period (usually 12 months) from the point at which the programme started. It can allude to a set amount of weight loss maintained, usually between 5–10 per cent, although as no clear definition has been agreed, in this book it refers to the maintenance of any amount of weight/fat lost.

Overweight – relating to an excess of body fat, regardless of weight.

Obesity – relating to a severe excess of body fat, regardless of weight, such that it increases the risk of disease. The term 'morbid obesity' is used occasionally to describe greatly increased risk of disease.

FOREWORD

Anybody who has tried to help overweight people achieve and maintain a healthy weight knows how difficult that is. Whether we are doctors, nurses, fitness professionals, counsellors or behaviour change specialists, most of us have struggled to persuade obese patients or clients to eat healthily and become physically active. Of course when they do it is hugely rewarding but personally I have often found it the most frustrating area in which to work, particularly when significant weight reduction is achieved only for it all to be put back on again in a few months!

If we are to be successful in helping people achieve and maintain a healthy weight then we must have a thorough understanding of obesity as an abnormal and unhealthy condition, what can be done about it and how to do it. This is what Paul Waters provides in this book. There is, of course, a plethora of books on obesity but few bring together such a breadth of information. It will be especially useful to fitness professionals, as increasingly we find ourselves working with overweight clients.

Paul approaches his subject in a clear and methodical manner. He explains complex physiology in a way that is accessible, easy to understand and with memorable illustrations. Paul is well known in the UK fitness sector for his teaching ability but what makes this book so useful is that he is also a practitioner. He has worked with many overweight clients, he knows what works and what does not. He has considerable insight into why clients find it so difficult to lose weight and why trainers find it so frustrating helping them to do so. But neither of these diminish his passion for wanting to assist clients in leading healthy lives because he knows from experience how transformative this can be.

This book is a mine of information and practical advice gathered into one volume. Paul has done clients and professionals alike a great service – in one form or another this book is an invaluable resource for those of us who work with overweight people.

Dr John Searle OBE
Formerly Honorary Chief Medical Officer ukactive
(formerly the Fitness Industry Association)

PREFACE

Read a newspaper, turn on the TV or go online today and you'll be hard-pressed not to see an article, story, advert or programme related to the worldwide issue of obesity. Health problems caused by being overweight, childhood obesity, the latest fad diet craze, new drugs or surgery that claim to offer a solution to the problem, research on nutrition, exercise, sleep, stress, or companies selling shakes or supplements touted as the miracle cure to the excess levels of fat that many of the world's population carry around with them every day.

In 2011, around 30 per cent of children in the UK were classified as overweight or obese (Public Health England, 2013). A recent news story based on a series of research papers suggested that by 2030, 48 per cent of British men and 42 per cent of British women will be classified as obese, with millions more overweight (NHS Choices, 2011). By 2050, it is estimated that 60 per cent of men, 50 per cent of women and 25 per cent of children will be obese (Public Health England, 2013). The picture in the USA is similar if not worse. In 2010, 36 per cent of adults were obese, that's around 85 million people, and a staggering 69 per cent, or 162 million were classified as overweight or obese (US Center for Disease Control and Prevention, 2011). This means that if a solution cannot be found, the definition of 'normal weight' will need to change dramatically, as being healthy will be considered unusual.

This book was borne out of a passion to help people to live healthier, happier lives and to help them to lose weight or to maintain a suitable weight for them in a healthy, sustainable way. This is not easy in the world we live in today. In recent years the world has been described as an 'obesogenic environment', where a whole host of factors have contributed towards the ever-expanding waistlines of the world's population, from the inhabitants of those warm islands of the South Pacific to the hardy indigenous tribes people who live high in the Arctic Circle.

The aim of this book is to link together all of the common threads in this oversized tapestry and give you an easy-to-follow guide as to the common causes of obesity and how changes in mindset, lifestyle, nutrition and exercise can help people to lose weight or keep it off in increasingly difficult circumstances. The advice given is based on scientific research and the wealth of experience gained in my many years in the fitness industry helping clients with their weight loss goals and listening to and working with instructors at the coalface. The book is addressed primarily to fitness and health professionals, but is written in such a way as to be easily read by anyone with an interest in the subject.

This is not another biased, one-sided or radical view on the 'best way to lose weight', a phrase often touted in magazines and online these days, but rather a resource for anyone interested in weight loss to refer to when needed. Weight loss works best with a holistic approach. As Aristotle once said 'the whole is greater than the sum of its parts', so the most effective weight loss and management can only be achieved through taking into account all of the elements contained in here. It is, however, perfectly possible to dip only into the single sections on goal setting and behaviour change, nutrition, exercise or lifestyle if these are the areas that you feel will be most beneficial.

Warn your clients (or yourself) not to expect the weight to disappear overnight, but help them to follow the principles of healthy living and they will find that it is possible to achieve a healthy weight and look the way they want to in the long term, without having to resort to another liquid diet, pill-popping experiment or six hour a day boot camp harder than most SAS training regimes.

I hope you find this book useful along the journey ahead and I hope that it helps a little towards making the world a happier, healthier, leaner place.

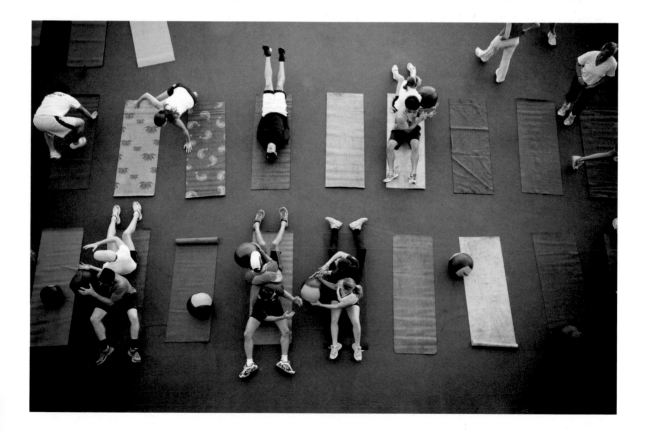

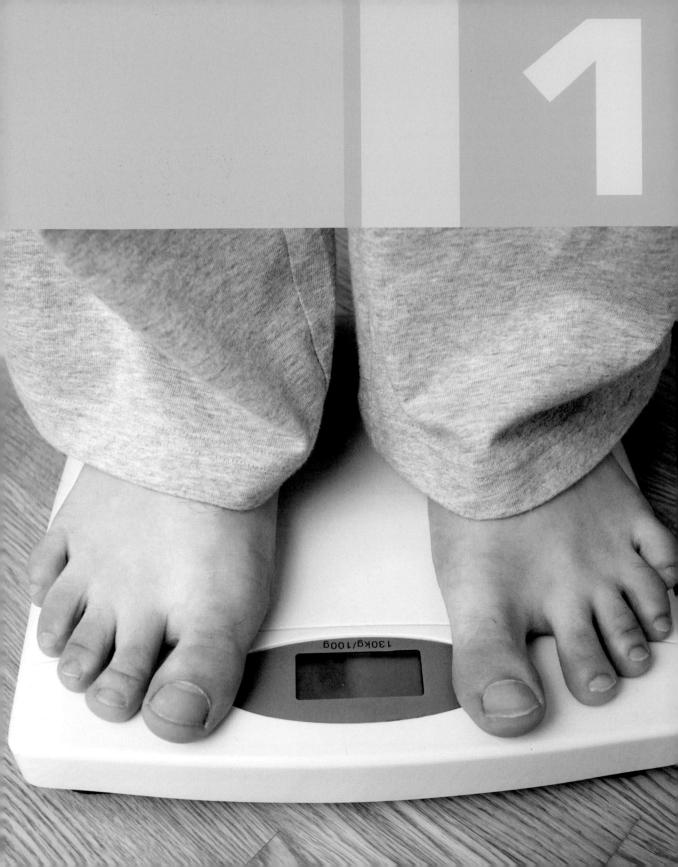

PART **ONE**

UNDERSTANDING WEIGHT GAIN AND WEIGHT LOSS

WEIGHTY MATTERS – THE WORLDWIDE OBESITY ISSUE

1

This chapter sets the scene for the book, identifying the size of the obesity problem at present, reviewing the numerous factors that help create the 'obesogenic' environment in which we live and highlighting the many illnesses that become more likely with weight gain.

BACKGROUND

Gallup Wellbeing® conducted a study recently showing that the self-reported weight of US men increased by around one and a half stone between 1990 and 2010 (Mendes, 2011), and this trend is consistent across the globe, with the UK no different. Clearly, something somewhere has gone wrong. The picture is the same the world over, with high levels of overweight and obese people to be found in almost every living civilisation on the planet.

So what exactly has led us down this path? It was, for a long time, put down to an imbalance in the energy equation, where calories consumed were greater than those burned. Although this does play a part, the answers to the question are far more complex and multifactorial, and can certainly not just be dismissed as being down to greed or laziness. They include:

- The technological age – with the invention of ever more machines that do what we once could only achieve with the sweat of our brows, life has, in essence, become easier. We no longer have to burn calories washing clothes or doing daily chores, we have numerous methods of transport that allow us to sit down to get almost anywhere in the world, our jobs have changed from those requiring hard labour to those needing only a seat, a desk and the ability move our fingers around a bit (an irony not lost on me as I sit here typing this). We can order our shopping online and have it delivered to our doorstep, and we do. The latest figures suggest that the Brits shop online more than any other nation in the world, spending £68 billion in 2011 (Hall, 2012).
- Television – OK, so this is part of the technological age, but it deserves its own special place in the list. The child of yesteryear spent most of their time out of school running around playing games, ranging from tag to hopscotch, skipping or football. Today's society prefers to watch others run around or, worse still, watch others do no exercise at all on their favourite reality TV show. When they do play games they tend to be on an Xbox or similar device,

controlling someone on screen who does the running around for them. Nintendo's Wii is at least a step (or swing of an imaginary tennis racket) in the right direction, but it is not enough on its own to stem the growing waistlines of the world's population.

• Food – or more importantly 'stuff that we are told is food' has changed dramatically over the past 50 years. In today's society it is increasingly difficult to eat 'naturally' and the prominence of heavily processed and refined foods; artificial ingredients like sweeteners and trans fats to add flavour and shelf life; and sugar, are overwhelming the bodies of adults and children. 'Real' food has become hard to get hold of and often only affordable to those higher up the social scale.

• Alcohol, drugs, lack of sleep, stress, some medications, fad diets, poor exercise advice and even our own genetic make-up all play significant roles in creating the 'obesogenic' environment that we now live in.

All of these risk factors plus more will be explained in greater detail later in this chapter. The idea that obesity is purely down to greed or laziness alone has been shown through a wealth of research not to be true. The intention here is certainly not to paint a bleak picture, rather it is to show the complex problem we face and to help you understand that there may be a number of things contributing to your clients' weight management challenges. Each of these are reviewed throughout the book so you will have a wealth of information at your fingertips to formulate a sensible, holistic approach to achieve long-lasting results. That said, you must emphasise to clients that weight loss is not easy and

requires sustained effort and permanent lifestyle changes to achieve and maintain.

THE (VERY) BIG PICTURE

Here are a couple of eye-opening stats:
• Obesity costs the NHS around £4.2 billion per year (Department of Health, 2011)
• In 2013, a two year-old boy became the youngest person ever to have weight loss surgery (Mail Online, 2013).

Obesity is interwoven into the very fabric of modern society. Clothing sizes have been steadily getting larger, it is impossible to watch an evening's television without seeing something on obesity, diet or health, adverts constantly deluge people with the new low-fat food or the best exercise routine. The media report daily on health and increasing waist sizes. Plane seats, chairs and hospital beds have been increasing in size and strength to cope with a heavier population, and TV shows such as *The Biggest Loser* or *Celebrity Fit Club* have popularised strict diet and exercise regimes.

RISK FACTORS
As you've already seen, there are a whole host of reasons why people have been gaining weight at an uncontrollable rate in the last generation. These can generally be classified as *modifiable* (things that can be controlled and changed) and *non-modifiable* (things that are beyond the control of the individual). There are always some grey areas when classifying things this way; for example,

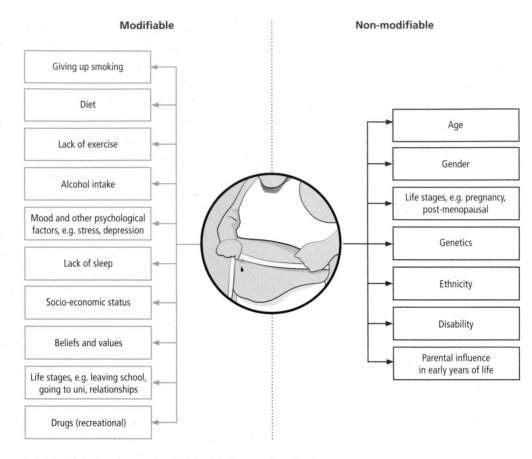

| Modifiable | | Non-modifiable |

Giving up smoking

Diet

Lack of exercise

Alcohol intake

Mood and other psychological factors, e.g. stress, depression

Lack of sleep

Socio-economic status

Beliefs and values

Life stages, e.g. leaving school, going to uni, relationships

Drugs (recreational)

Age

Gender

Life stages, e.g. pregnancy, post-menopausal

Genetics

Ethnicity

Disability

Parental influence in early years of life

Figure 1.1 Modifiable and non-modifiable risk factors for obesity

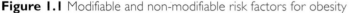

a life stress may not be possible to remove from someone's life, such as a close family member being ill, but the response to that stress may be managed to improve their response to this.

It is important for you to know the underlying mechanisms of how these risk factors bring about weight gain. You should be able to explain these to your clients in language that is simple to understand and relates to their goals. The following information is designed to help you with this. The relevant chapters then provide you with information about the changes that people can make to

lose weight and positively impact their health at the same time. Let's first look at the modifiable risk factors.

MODIFIABLE RISK FACTORS
NUTRITION

Arguably one of the largest risk factors for weight gain, or more specifically for increases in body fat, is the food that we eat. As mentioned earlier, it is not just the over consumption of calories that plays a part, although clearly this is a factor.

Quality of food is essential, with the wrong choices causing a cascade of events that affect hormone levels, putting the body into 'storage mode' and saving those extra calories consumed for a rainy day. How and when the body stores fat is reviewed in more detail in Chapter 2 and the foods that are the worst offenders for bringing this about are detailed in Chapter 5.

EXERCISE AND ACTIVITY

In simple terms, the lack of daily movement is a major contributing factor to increased body fat. If we don't burn the calories off then we end up with more than we need and, rather than let them go to waste, the body decides that it might be a good idea to hold on to them, just in case we have to go without food for a long time. This is part of our evolutionary design and arguably one of the biggest reasons for our survival. Up until relatively recently in our history, we may have spent some time without substantial amounts of food available. In winter, when food was scarce, we could then dip into our body fat stores if required. The problem that most of us in modern society have today is that we have constant access to an abundance of calories. We don't have to go foraging or hunting for food, we merely put our coats on, drive to the local supermarket, buy a ready meal, drive home and pop it in the microwave while we settle down to watch *EastEnders*.

Another significant factor exercise plays is in maintaining muscle mass, or *lean mass* as it is sometimes called. Muscle uses a lot of energy and good levels of muscle stoke the furnace within us and help keep us lean. As we age, unless we stay active, our muscle mass decreases and with it our ability to burn calories. You don't have to look like Arnold Schwarzenegger to burn calories effectively but keeping a moderate degree of lean mass can be of huge benefit in the battle against middle-age spread.

Finally, exercise helps to balance all of those hormones that you'll read more about in Chapter 2. These little things drive our appetites and how and when we store and burn fat, so can have a strong bearing on how lean we remain.

LACK OF SLEEP

Think about it; if you want to keep a fire burning for longer, you need to put more logs on it. Similarly, if you're awake for longer, your body thinks it needs more fuel to keep it going. Studies show that a lack of sleep increases the levels of an important hormone called *ghrelin* (Taheri et al, 2004; Spiegel et al, 2004), one that drives us to feel hungry. Coupled with this, tiredness generally leads to poor food choices, reaching for high-energy processed foods to give us that boost we're after. The trouble is, if we're tired and not exercising as much as we should, we don't burn this off, instead we store it as fat. In fact, these high-energy snacks cause our blood sugars to rise and then crash soon after as our bodies battle to deal with the rush of energy. We quickly feel hungry and tired again and repeat the cycle many times across the day. You'll read more about this later when we look at glycaemic index and glycaemic load in Chapter 5.

ALCOHOL

Alcohol achieves notoriety as being one of the few substances to act as both a stimulant and a depressant. It stimulates blood glucose to rise while at the same time dulling the responses of the central nervous system.

It may not be surprising to know that consuming too much alcohol can lead to weight gain, but it may surprise you as to the number of different ways in which it brings this about. Alcohol contains calories and, just like calories from other sources, these can be stored away as fat if they're not used. Many alcoholic drinks are also high in sugar and can affect blood glucose levels. This brings about the same cycle of events mentioned above. Blood sugars will rise and fall when we reach for unhealthy food choices, store them away and then do it again shortly afterwards. Think about the food you ate the last time you had a hangover – I'd be surprised if it was grilled fish and vegetables.

GIVING UP SMOKING

If you, or your client, are giving up, or packed up recently, then firstly well done! Quitting smoking is one of the best things that can be done for

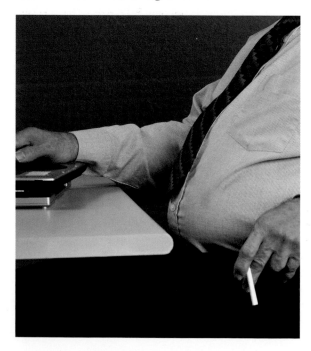

health, and research now shows that giving up at any age can improve health and extend lifespan. Even those who quit at 60 can add another three years to their lives (NHS Choices, 2012).

One of the challenges of giving up smoking is that nicotine suppresses appetite. Many find that quitting leads them to gain weight shortly afterwards. Firstly, let's point out that not smoking and being a few pounds heavier is still arguably better for health than being lighter and filling the body with toxins and chemicals on a daily basis. That said, it's likely that some of your clients may not see it this way. But it is possible to pack in without snackin'. The key to staying light without lighting up appears to lie in controlling blood sugars. We've touched on this already and it will be a constant theme throughout this book. Eating low glycaemic load foods (see Chapter 5 for more details) and balancing meals by combining carbohydrates with protein can help control appetite.

Smokers also say that when they give up they are used to holding something in their hands and in many cases, to beat the signals from the brain urging them to smoke, they replace cigarettes with food. Chapter 7 shows how you can help your clients by ensuring they have healthy snacks to hand instead of biscuits, crisps and chocolate bars.

STRESS AND OTHER PSYCHOLOGICAL FACTORS

Food and mood are inextricably linked. Even the healthiest person has been known to reach for the ice cream in times of stress, anger, anxiety or upset. This is because food is, in reality, a very powerful drug, altering levels of hormones in the body that, for a short while at least, provide pleasure or relaxation. Real foods can have a positive impact on chemicals in the body, but the heavily processed and refined stuff, which arguably isn't food at all, can wreak havoc and create a hormonal soup that is perfect for promoting fat storage. This, coupled with the fact that hormones are already on a rollercoaster ride when stressed, can lead to a habit of reaching for 'comfort foods' whenever the mood takes hold.

SOCIAL FACTORS AND LIFE STAGES

A person's social life can have a major impact on their weight and health. Some spend their time with friends going for a run, playing tennis or rock climbing, while others meet up in the local pub.

Diet and activity are strongly influenced by what is going on in a person's life at the time. There are a number of life stages when a person's risk for weight gain is increased. The ones that can be controlled, or where the person's lifestyle can be managed, are:

- Leaving school
- Going to university
- Relationships
- Life changes such as a new job or moving house

BELIEFS AND VALUES

This is challenging territory. Working with clients to alter their beliefs or values takes skill and you can encounter many obstacles along the way. So what are beliefs and values? Ready and Burton (2010, p.44) describe them in the following way. Beliefs are 'the generalisations made about life experiences', while values are described as 'the "hot buttons" that drive all of your behaviours'. In essence, beliefs are the things you hold to be true and values are the things that are important to you.

People's beliefs and values can be deep-seated and formed over many years. Changing them can literally be life changing and equivalent to lifting up their house in suburban England and plonking it back down in the middle of the Sahara dessert. It takes a lot of effort for a person to adapt to their new outlook on life and can be a reason why many people fall off the wagon when losing weight, or even after they have achieved their goals. Let's look at a few examples:

CASE STUDY 1

A client, Geoff, had no desire to reduce his alcohol intake, even though he was overweight and his blood tests showed that his liver was no longer functioning as it should. When questioned about his reasons for not wanting to change, he explained that his father had been advised to give up alcohol by his doctor. He did so but a few months later he died of a heart attack. Geoff believed that giving up alcohol had brought this about, as this was the one thing his father had changed. When discussing this, Geoff was asked to consider the possibility that the two may have been unrelated or that his father may have given up too late, the effects of his years of drinking being a possible factor. He was open to the idea and embarked on a healthier lifestyle with greatly reduced alcohol intake. A number of months later when he returned for another check-up, he had lost a considerable amount of weight, his liver function had improved and, more importantly, his belief that giving up alcohol was bad for your health had been changed.

CASE STUDY 2

Another client, Lidia, was struggling to lose weight. She said she had been trying for some time but no matter what she did, exercising more and generally being healthier, she hadn't lost any and her clothes sizes remained the same. When talking through the possible reasons for this she said she could not think of any. We talked about her lifestyle in general and she went through her daily routines. After a while she mentioned her daughter and the fact that she had previously been anorexic but was now recovering. She admitted that when her daughter was around she would often eat in an attempt to encourage her to do so as well. She identified that she did this even when she was full and would often consume larger portions at dinner. She hadn't realised she was doing this and when asked what she could do about it she said she would talk to her daughter to explain that she wanted to lose weight and reach a healthy body fat percentage. Her daughter was very supportive and between them they worked out an eating pattern that was healthy for both of them. As Lidia's daughter was so important to her in her values, she had subconsciously been focusing on her needs rather than her own. Once she recognised this and worked out a way to continue caring for her daughter while at the same time looking after her own health she was able to make the changes she needed. Within two months she had lost nearly a stone in weight and a number of inches from her waist.

GUT BACTERIA

Yes, you read that correctly. It has been proposed that the bacteria in the digestive system may have a role to play in either people becoming obese, or in their ability to lose weight once gained. There are two main types of gut bacteria, Bacteroidetes and Firmicutes. When you gain weight, the balance of the two is changed, possibly altering the amount of energy that can be stored (Turnbaugh et al, 2006). At present this is far from conclusive, but it is clear that a healthy diet can play a part in ensuring a good balance of gut bacteria (Duncan et al, 2008). It appears this is because certain foods like fruits, vegetables and live yoghurt contain prebiotics and probiotics, substances that, when consumed, help create more healthy bacteria in the gut. It is this information that has led to the huge rise in the number of probiotic drinks available on the market. While there is clear evidence for the benefits of probiotics for relief from diarrhoea and to support those taking antibiotics, whose 'good bacteria' can be destroyed by the drugs, research is still needed on other possible health benefits and the actual content of certain bacteria within some drinks has been questioned (Scheinbach, 1998). They don't appear to do any harm but, as mentioned, fruit, vegetables and live yoghurt will help increase the healthy bacteria regardless.

DRUGS

This may not apply to a lot of people but it is well worth mentioning the powerful effects that recreational drugs can have on body fat levels and health. Using marijuana, or coming off it, may result in changes in appetite and eating behaviour for some, which could lead to weight gain (Mohs et al, 1990). Of course, some may have to take some type of drug, in the form of medication, which brings us nicely to the non-modifiable risk factors.

NON-MODIFIABLE RISK FACTORS
MEDICATION

Many medications work by altering levels of various substances inside the human body. This often helps to manage or improve the symptoms of the ailment from which a person is suffering but can also bring about other unwanted changes – one of the common side effects being weight gain. While it's not precisely clear why this happens, it may be to do with changes in levels of hormones, metabolic rate and appetite brought about by the drugs. Very commonly used medications such as the contraceptive pill, antidepressants or corticosteroids (anti-inflammatories, not the bodybuilding type) can lead to increased fat stores.

AGE

Obviously people can't change their age. Ageing brings about changes in the body and from surprisingly early on in life. Muscle and bone mass unless stimulated by exercise will start to decrease from about 35 years old. As muscle mass decreases so does metabolic rate, and the body becomes less effective at burning calories. This leads to gradual gains in body fat until the dreaded middle-age spread takes hold shortly afterwards.

Of course, while this process is associated with ageing, and people can't travel back in time, regular exercise can offset the effects of ageing – meaning that it is possible to manage the risk to an extent.

The effects of ageing on women specifically are covered more below in relation to the impact of the menopause.

GENDER

Men are from Mars, women are from Venus – or so the saying goes. In relation to the storage of fat, it is the hormones within our bodies that make us so different. Women have high levels of oestrogen and progesterone while men have high levels of testosterone, aldosterone and androgen. These differences affect where we store our fat, how much lean muscle we have and a host of other factors relating to weight loss and gain.

Women tend to predominantly store fat around their hips, thighs and the backs of their arms, while men are more likely to carry it on their back and around their waist. Changes in diet, exercise and hormone levels can alter this, but in general a man's increased risk of heart disease stems from the fact that they tend to be more 'apple-shaped', carrying a 'spare tyre' around their middle. This fat is known as *visceral fat* as it sits between the internal organs (viscera), where it can interfere with normal functions and increase the risk of disease. It had been thought until recently that

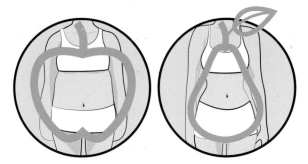

Figure 1.2 Apples and pears: the different body shapes by fat storage location

women were at decreased risk of heart disease and other conditions because they are more 'pear-shaped', but some studies have suggested to the contrary (Jialal et al, 2013).

LIFE STAGE

Some stages of life, such as going to university, were classified as modifiable risk factors earlier in this chapter due to the fact that the individual can control their environment. Others, however, are partly or completely beyond the control of the individual. These include early childhood, pregnancy and the menopause.

Very young children have little or no say in how active they are or what they are given to eat by their parents. This can have a substantial bearing on obesity in later life, with studies reporting that gaining weight in the formative years impacts size later in childhood and possibly beyond (Ong and Loos, 2007).

During pregnancy and menopause, a range of hormonal changes including altered levels of oestrogen, progesterone and stress hormones, cause multiple changes throughout the body, including alteration of appetite and can increase the risk for weight gain. While the effects of this can be controlled, the changes in the hormones themselves cannot.

GENETICS

Is there any truth that a person's weight, shape and body fat levels are all in their genes? Or is the size of their jeans all down to them? Over the past 20 years or so, scientists have identified hundreds of genes that play a part in regulating weight, including 50 since 2006 (Centers for Disease Control, 2013). What the research has shown, as you will see in more detail in Chapter 2, is that all of these genes can account for only a percentage of a person's fat levels. This means that, while they do certainly play a part, it is not inevitable that if you have 'the wrong genes' (a yet to be made adaptation of a Wallace and Gromit film adventure), you are doomed to live a life battling the bulge.

Of course, people naturally come in all shapes and sizes. They can generally be classified as one of three main body types:

- Ectomorph
- Endomorph
- Mesomorph

Ectomorphs are generally small-framed with narrow hips and waist, the 'beanpole' physique as it is often unkindly referred to. Ectomorphs are typically seen in sports like long-distance running where their light frames are more suited to the high mileage required. They can find it difficult to gain muscle and certainly, in their younger years, they are often the person who seems able to eat what they like without gaining a pound. They sometimes fool themselves later in life that they are healthy because they are small, although this has now been shown not to be true. Some ectomorphs can have high levels of body fat, especially internal fat sitting around their organs, but at the same time look thin to their friends and relatives when clothed. If they have high internal fat they are at just as big a risk of heart disease as someone who is outwardly fatter.

Endomorphs are generally larger framed and can gain fat far more easily than their ectomorph counterparts. Endomorphs can lose weight – as can anyone on the planet – if they address the issues outlined in this book, but they may find it more of a challenge and certainly will not change their body shape completely. Endomorphs don't become ectomorphs, rather they become leaner endomorphs; as one of my lecturers at university used to say: 'You can make a Shire horse a faster Shire horse, but you can't turn it into a racehorse.'

Mesomorphs are naturally muscular, to the envy of many of their friends, certainly the males. They may never have seen a weight in a gym, but seemingly carry a good amount of muscle mass nonetheless. If they ever do train they find they can bulk up with relative ease when compared to the ectomorph who strives so hard to gain the tiniest amount of muscle (your author is one of the latter and has gained a reasonable muscle tone through 12 years of training but will never be Arnold Schwarzenegger).

People can be a combination of these body types, for example someone may be a meso-endo and gain fat and muscle easily, some rugby players are good examples of this type. Ecto-mesos are generally lean and muscular, the envy of many and destined to be cover models for July's edition of *Men's Fitness*.

There are some medical conditions created by genetic defects that put people at a greatly increased risk of weight gain. These include:

- Prader Willi syndrome
- Bardet-Biedl syndrome
- Alstrom syndrome
- Cohen syndrome

Prader Willi in particular has hit the headlines in recent years and affects around one in 15,000 people. Sufferers have a genetic defect that makes them feel extremely hungry. This may be connected to changes in levels of the hormone leptin, although studies differ on this. Prader Willi sufferers may often have associated challenges with learning, emotions and behaviour, and it is not uncommon for them to become violent if deprived of constant access to food. They can become overweight at a very young age and in

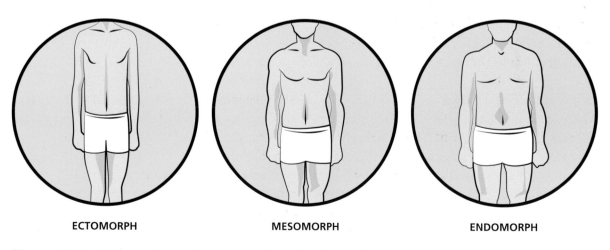

ECTOMORPH   MESOMORPH   ENDOMORPH

Figure 1.3 Body types: ectomorphs, mesomorphs and endomorphs

some instances end up in care as their parents struggle to cope. Even if living at home, they will have an assigned health care worker who can assist the parents in managing the day-to-day challenges of restricting food access and intake, as well as the accompanying mood swings.

Bardet-Biedl, Alstrom and Cohen syndrome are all very rare conditions, with Alstrom syndrome in particular only affecting a few hundred people worldwide. All are caused by gene mutations and can have a wide range of effects on sufferers, weight gain being just one.

ETHNICITY

Like gender and age, ethnicity is clearly not something that can be changed but it can have a bearing on fat stores and risk for disease. Asian populations may for instance have much higher risk of developing type 2 diabetes, with Hispanic populations and Afro-Caribbeans at a higher risk than Caucasians (Harvard School of Public Health, 2013), although there is some debate as to how much of this is down to ethnicity and how much relates to culture and lifestyle. Ethnicity clearly has some bearing on size and shape, with the average build of a South Pacific islander substantially different to that of a Chinese person.

OTHER CONDITIONS

There are other illnesses or conditions that may increase the risk of obesity. Those with physical disabilities may be at increased risk as their ability to move and burn calories can be limited. Illnesses such as type 2 diabetes will inhibit the metabolic function of the body, making it challenging to lose weight. An underactive thyroid does the same, as it means decreased levels of thyroxine, the hormone that drives energy production and therefore calorie

burn. An overactive thyroid, however, can lead to weight loss even when appetite is normal.

Can you catch obesity?

In recent years it has been proposed by some scientists that viruses may cause weight gain. Studies on animals have identified a range of potential viral causes, and in humans the Ad-36 Adenovirus has been linked. In studies on twins, those exposed to the virus were heavier and fatter than their sibling (Atkinson, 2007). It appears that Ad-36 has an impact on a number of cellular and enzymatic processes within the body, increasing the fat stores as a consequence. Other viruses have also been linked to weight gain including SMAM-1, common in birds (Vasilakopoulou and le Roux, 2007).

RISK OF ILLNESS

While many things can increase the risk of gaining weight, equally being overweight or obese brings with it an increased risk for developing a huge range of medical conditions, including but not limited to:

- Diabetes type 2
- Sleep apnoea
- Certain cancers including colon, prostate and stomach
- Gallstones
- Kidney and liver problems
- Heart attack
- Stroke
- High blood pressure (hypertension)
- High cholesterol
- Other cardiovascular disease

In fact, being obese increases the risk of some cancers by as much as 40 per cent (National Cancer Institute, 2012). A 5 per cent decrease in body weight can cut the risk of type 2 diabetes in half (Diabetes Prevention Program Research Group, 2002) and men who are not obese but merely overweight (BMI 25–29.9) have been shown to have a 72 per cent increased risk for developing heart disease (Eckel, 1997).

SUMMARY

- Obesity has reached epidemic proportions across the globe.
- There are a vast range of risk factors responsible, some of which are modifiable and some that are not. While genetics plays its part for some, improvements in weight can be made.
- Obesity increases the risk for a wide range of diseases.

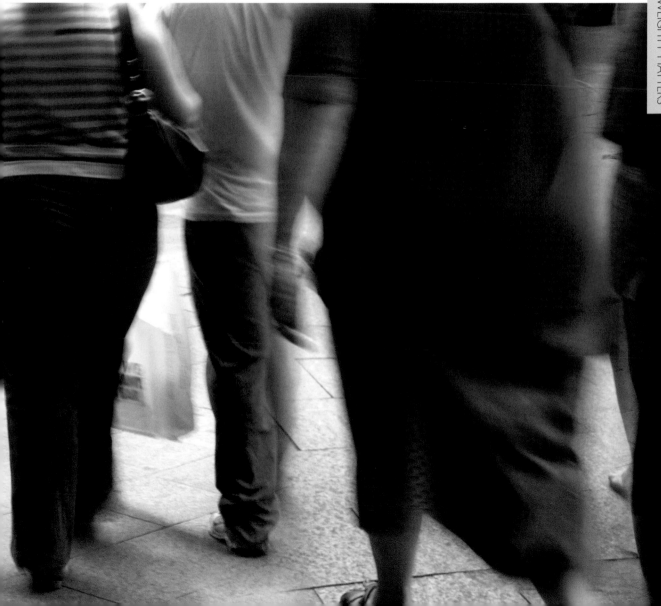

HOW THE BODY REGULATES WEIGHT 2

This chapter takes a simple look at the mechanisms the body has to control weight, fat storage and fat burning. It looks at what metabolism is, how it works and how it may be estimated for an individual, as well as identifying organs, hormones and neurotransmitters that play a role in appetite, energy storage and production.

METABOLISM

Everybody has heard the word metabolism, indeed many put their weight gain down to the fact that theirs must be 'slow'. Research now shows that this is not the case for most; indeed, as people gain weight their metabolic rate increases to cope with having to carry their extra weight around. So just what is metabolism?

In simple terms, it is all of the energy burning and cell-building activities that the body goes through on a daily basis. Metabolism is made of two components:

- *Anabolism*: from ancient Greek, meaning 'throw up', it involves all of the cell-building processes including muscle building, regrowth of tissues, hair and everything else that degenerates and rebuilds many times over the course of a lifetime.

- *Catabolism*: from ancient Greek, meaning 'throw down', it includes all of the processes that break down energy or tissues including the use of carbohydrates and fats for exercise, the breakdown of muscle protein to produce energy in times of need and all of the breaking down and clearing away of old or damaged cells over time.

Put simply:

Anabolism + Catabolism = Metabolism

Those who want to gain muscle mass need to be in an anabolic state, that is, building up more than they are breaking down so that they can achieve their goal of increased muscle size. It is logical then that people who want to lose weight need to be in a catabolic state, right? Well, yes and no. This has been the downfall of many a person trying to 'lose weight' or, in reality, to reduce stores of fat. Catabolism is required to lose weight but an anabolic state where enough muscle is maintained is also important. If you asked most people what their weight loss goal was they would be unlikely to say 'Oh yeah, I'm just too muscular and want to get rid of that lean, toned look I've got.' The truth is that, for the majority of people, when then say 'weight loss' they mean they want to look leaner, smaller and more toned. Ask your clients if they looked the way they wanted to but didn't know what they weighed would they be happy? Many reply with a resounding yes. It's about how their clothes fit or how they look to their partner in that dress or on the beach.

Losing 'weight' requires decreasing body fat levels and the way to do this effectively *is to build or maintain lean muscle mass*. Muscle burns more calories at rest than fat does. It is also denser and as such takes up less space, decreasing waistline and clothing size. Many people are surprised by how heavy some very lean individuals such as athletes are, even though they are in great shape.

So how do you know just how much energy a person requires to function? Resting Metabolic Rate (RMR) is a measure of how many calories the body requires per day to stay the same weight. This is slightly different to Basal Metabolic Rate (BMR), which is a measure of the minimum amount of calories required by the body for essential functions like breathing to occur. The most accurate way to measure this is to monitor someone inside a specially created living chamber that measures daily energy intake and expenditure, although these are only found in science labs and not widely accessible to the general public. This is discussed in more detail later on. There are various calculations that have been put forward to work out RMR. The simplest of these is:

Weight (kg) × 25 = RMR (kcals*)

* *Kcals is a term commonly substituted for calories*

For example, an 80 kg person would have an RMR of 2,000 kcals per day.

80 × 25 = 2,000.

This is great but the reality is that most people don't just sit completely still all day (well, maybe lots of them do – and that's why this book is needed!). To get a more accurate measure of someone's daily calorie requirement you need to know how active the person is. See the table below to work out total daily calorie needs:

Table 2.1	Daily calorie needs
Activity Level	**Multiplication of RMR**
Sedentary (mostly inactive, desk-based job)	1.2
Moderately active (moderate intensity exercise 3–5 days per week)	1.5
Very active (physical job + frequently active or following athlete training schedule)	2.0

As an example, if our 80 kg person were sedentary they'd have a daily calorie requirement of 2,400.

80 × 25 = 2,000 × 1.2 = 2,400

This calorie intake would, in theory, mean that they would maintain their weight over time. Alternatively, if they were very active the calculation would be as follows:

80 × 25 = 2,000 × 2 = 4,000

As you can see, the level of activity makes a substantial difference to how many calories a person needs on a daily basis to maintain weight.

This calculation is only an *estimate* of metabolism. There are many others, such as the Harris-Benedict, Schofield, and Katch and McArdle equations, the last of which is discussed in more detail shortly. The Schofield equation takes into account height and weight, while the Katch and McArdle calculation also uses lean mass, making it possibly the most accurate of all due to its impact on calorie use.

IS IT REALLY THAT SIMPLE?

Unfortunately, no. If it was, it's likely that we wouldn't find ourselves facing the challenge we do today, as people would have discovered their 'magic number' and have used this as their daily target to ensure they lost those excess pounds.

There are a couple of reasons complicating this:

1. Not all people who weigh the same have the same calorie requirements.
2. Not all calories are equal.

As you've already seen, muscle and fat act very differently on the body. Muscle is far more metabolically active and as such requires a lot more calories than an equal amount of fat to sustain it. Two people both weighing 80 kg could have very different calorific requirements if one had 10 per cent body fat and the other had 30 per cent body fat. The leaner individual could actually devour more calories without gaining weight, as their body would be more capable of burning them off. It's kind of like having two cars that weigh the same; one's a 1.1 litre runaround for your grandma and the other is a 2.0 litre turbo engine Japanese sports car. Although they weigh the same, they have very different fuel consumption.

Up until recent times, it was believed that all calories were equal and that it was about how much you put inside you that was the defining factor in weight loss and weight gain. There is now growing research into the effects that different nutrients have on the body and it offers interesting insights into the idea that counting calories may not add up; in this case one plus one may not equal two.

This may be because the body treats 'natural food' very differently than it does highly processed refined sugars and fats. In nature, foods don't contain high quantities of sugar and fat together and so our caveman bodies never experienced high levels of both sugar and fat in the bloodstream at the same time. This modern mixture can be problematic as it essentially promotes fat storage; it does so because the burst of sugar raises insulin levels in response to the higher than normal levels. Insulin, in turn, causes the body to store energy and it just so happens that there's a whole load of fat swimming around ready to be stored.

Eat a piece of fish and some vegetables and, while the body will still store excess energy if short-term energy stores are already full, the same dramatic fat storing response won't occur. This will be looked at in more detail in relation to hormones later in this chapter and the section on glycaemic load and glycaemic index in Chapter 5. Here you'll get some useful insight in how to manage diet to minimise fat gains.

BETTER MATHS

Some calculations used to estimate metabolic rate might be better than others, although there is still debate around which to use. The Katch and McArdle Formula (McArdle et al, 2010) takes into account not only weight but also lean mass. As we've seen, muscle is more metabolically active and so it makes sense to include this variable in a calculation. Their formula is as follows:

$$BMR = 370 + (21.6 \times lean\ mass\ (kg))$$

So if two people both weighed 80 kg, but one had a lean mass of 72 kg (10 per cent body fat) and the other had a lean mass of 60 kg (25 per cent body fat) their BMRs would be:

10 per cent body fat: 1,915 kcals
25 per cent body fat: 1,671 kcals

As you can see the leaner individual requires nearly 250 kcals per day more just to function normally. The actual daily calorie requirements could be calculated using the table on page 15.

Even so, this is still only an estimate. The most accurate ways of measuring energy expenditure include direct calorimetry and the doubly labelled water technique. Both are highly scientific and not practical for everyday use but provide valuable information to scientists about how the body expends energy. I have included details about each of them in the box above.

While it's interesting to know how the scientists do it, calorie intake does not always have to be measured to achieve weight loss. Some may not want to count calories all day or make it a part of their everyday lives in the long term. They may be successful by simply changing their diet or increasing the amount they exercise. If you do use calculations of calorie requirements with clients, their weight multiplied by 25 is the simplest method but

Measuring energy expenditure

Direct calorimetry measures a person's use of oxygen and exhalation of carbon dioxide, or other measures such as changes in air or water temperature by placing them in a specially designed chamber – basically a room with equipment for measuring changes in the make-up of the atmosphere. The subject can live in there for a period of time, eating, watching TV or exercising. From the measures taken, calculations can estimate calorie expenditure.

Doubly labelled water experiments involve subjects drinking special water, containing a radioisotope, a radioactive but ultimately non-harmful element, which can be tracked as it enters and leaves the body. From this, carbon dioxide production can be calculated and, in turn, oxygen consumption. The measures take place over a period of about three weeks and, while it is useful for measuring energy expenditure over time, the test is impractical and extremely expensive.

may not be very accurate. The Katch and McArdle option offers better accuracy but can be a little more time-consuming. You'll need to recalculate regularly based on changes in lean mass and activity levels.

HORMONES AND GLANDS

Hormones are chemicals that the body creates to send messages around the body. They are capable of switching things on and off or speeding up and slowing down bodily functions. Adrenaline, for example, will speed up heart rate and breathing rate among other things when you need to run away from something. Glands are the things in the body, often organs, which produce hormones.

WHY DO WE HAVE THEM?

Your body works best when it is in *homeostasis*, or normal, balanced functioning. There are times though when it needs to work faster and others when it needs to slow down. Hormones are triggers that switch things on or off, speed up or slow down things like heart rate, and increase or decrease levels of things like blood sugar, dependent on what the body needs. Ideally the body will work in a balanced way, so it will be down as much as it is up and off as much as it is on. The right balance of hormones helps this to happen.

HOW DO THEY AFFECT WEIGHT LOSS AND GAIN?

Hormones have many roles in the body and a number are involved in the production and storage of energy, the regulation of appetite and in helping the body release energy when needed to for movement and exercise. These all have a bearing on how much fat a person stores at any one time and how much weight they lose or gain. The main hormones you should be aware of are identified below.

INSULIN AND GLUCAGON

These two hormones, insulin in particular, play a major part in the storage of fat within the body. They are effectively complete opposites and should work together to regulate blood sugars up and down when required to keep your body functioning normally.

Glucagon is released when blood sugars drop. This may occur if someone has not eaten for a while or has exercised and their blood sugar levels have decreased as a result. Glucagon is released by the pancreas and through a chain of events causes the liver to release the body's store of glucose (known as glycogen) into the bloodstream. This elevates blood sugar levels and enables the person to function properly.

In evolutionary terms, glucagon was a very useful hormone as it was needed in times of 'fight or flight' to elevate blood sugar levels. It also came into play if a person went a while without food. The brain needs a steady supply of energy, so if it couldn't be supplied by food, the body was able to dip into its back-up stores to increase blood sugars and give the brain the fuel it required. We have maintained all of these evolutionary functions and they are still useful in today's world, although in Western society it is very rare for people to go any length of time without access to any food at all.

It has not been shown that any discrepancies in glucagon levels bring about obesity, but it does appear that in overweight individuals glucagon may not be as effective at raising energy usage as in normal weight people (Starke et al, 1984).

Insulin is one of the most important hormones when it comes to weight gain and associated medical conditions, especially diabetes. It has a number of jobs but its major role is to decrease blood sugars if they get too high. These days this can happen a lot with our highly processed and refined high-sugar diets. Each time a person consumes a chocolate bar, some white bread or a can of fizzy drink, insulin is called into action as the level of glucose in the blood soars above what is required. The body responds by pulling this glucose out of the bloodstream and into storage just in case it needs it later. If stores of sugars are full then, instead of wasting it, the body converts it to fat, and stores it.

If this happens regularly over time, the body becomes less sensitive to the insulin and blood sugars will stay high. In response to this, the body releases more insulin to get the desired response. This keeps happening until the body becomes extremely insensitive to insulin and blood sugars remain high most of the time. This is type 2 diabetes. It can get even worse; if the poor lifestyle persists, the pancreas gets exhausted from having to produce so much insulin and effectively gives in. These later-stage diabetics aren't just insensitive to insulin, they often don't produce any and rely on injections to get what they need and help their body regulate its blood sugar levels. Coupled with this, the high levels of glucose can cause damage throughout the body and weight control becomes extremely challenging.

It has been argued by some that the insulin response and the body's subsequent insensitivity are the major factors in the obesity epidemic (Taubes, 2013). This argument is commonly used in many of the high-fat, high-protein, low-carb diets that have been popular over the last 20 years that are reviewed in more detail in Chapter 5. There is a growing support for higher-fat diets in science, especially for those people with diabetes where low-carb diets may improve insulin sensitivity and reduce the subsequent risks. Guldbrand et al (2012) showed that over two years a low-carbohydrate diet containing 50 per cent fat and 20 per cent carbohydrate led to a significant drop in blood sugars in diabetic patients, allowing them to reduce their insulin medication. This was not seen in a group consuming 60 per cent carbohydrates and 30 per cent fat as per current government recommendations. Marshall

and Bessesen (2002), however, argue the opposite, noting that many studies suggest that high-fat diets are shown to impair insulin function – and so the debate rages on.

LEPTIN AND GHRELIN

Along with insulin, another hormone that has received huge attention in recent years in relation to fat storage is leptin. It is produced mostly by the fat cells themselves and its job is to tell someone when they're full. The opposing hormone, ghrelin, is made in the stomach when it is empty and tells someone when he or she is hungry. Together these hormones talk to the hypothalamus in the brain to regulate when and how much to eat. But if something goes wrong or they become unbalanced then gains in fat stores may be just around the corner as the fat-storing tendencies of the body and a person's appetite are increased.

It used to be assumed that as people ate more their leptin levels increased and appetite was suppressed. This is certainly what should happen, but research has shown that if someone consumes too many calories and gains weight, they can become leptin resistant in much the same way they can become resistant to insulin. What this means is that 'fullness' signals don't get through and someone is far more likely to keep eating. Myers, Cowley and Munzberg (2008) showed that leptin resistance is caused by a number of complex factors, including changes in chemical process and changes in signalling between cells, with the end result being increased hunger and weight gain.

In contrast, when losing weight the body reacts by decreasing leptin and raising levels of ghrelin, increasing hunger. This may be a very influential factor in the reason why so many that lose weight gain much or all of it back, and sometimes more on top. It has been suggested that rapid dieting may make this worse and increase the likelihood that all of the hard work will be undone. Some argue that a more gradual weight loss may help to prevent this and allow the body to gradually adapt to its new weight without reacting and bouncing back to its original start point as is seen in diets where rapid weight loss occurs (Amigo and Fernandez, 2007).

Linked to this is the notion of the Set Point Theory. While the precise origin of this theory is difficult to pin down, various researchers have studied or made reference to it (Weinsier et al, 2000; Pereira et al, 2004). The theory suggests that a person's weight is genetically predetermined, and that, should they diet, their body will increase various signals, including ghrelin levels, to ramp up hunger. This makes weight regain likely and research certainly shows that this is common. Wing and Phelan (2005) suggest that only around 20 per cent of people maintain weight loss after one year if losing 10 per cent or more of their original body weight.

Set Point Theory has always been controversial and arguments have swung back and forth between those who believe genetics leads to weight gain and those who believe it is due to poor diet or a lack of exercise. In reality, it is likely that both are true – with people having a weight and body fat that they would likely be naturally, but that today's environment including poor food and sedentary lifestyles can drive people away from their natural set point to a higher level, resetting the set point and making it difficult to return to 'normal' (Müller et al, 2010).

Remember, you've already seen that people are 'naturally' different in Chapter 1 when looking at ectomorphs, endomorphs and mesomorphs.

STRESS HORMONES

The body has a number of hormones that are activated in times of stress, including adrenaline and cortisol. These are known as 'fight or flight' hormones, and are raised by:

- Physical stress – this includes positive stress such as exercise, but also negative stresses such as fighting off an attacker or running away from a dangerous dog.
- Mental stress – people don't have to run away from something for their stress hormones to be activated. Tight work deadlines and stressful jobs are commonplace these days, arguments with friends and family, financial worries and a host of other reasons will send stress hormones soaring.
- Hunger – this may surprise you but hunger is a physical stress on the body. That's why it releases ghrelin to drive people to eat; otherwise it can't function properly. It's even worse if people ignore these signals and don't eat. High levels of ghrelin are also linked to increased adrenaline in the blood with the body getting stressed as it knows that the low blood sugar levels and empty stomach it has identified mean that soon the brain won't have the supply of energy it needs to work effectively. The rise in adrenaline causes the liver to release stores of glucagon (stored carbohydrate) and blood sugars return to normal without having to eat. Of course this means that the back-up stores are now running low, so eating is essential to keep them maintained.
- In fact a stress is really anything that requires the body to move away from homeostasis, its normal state. This can include changes in temperature, chemical levels in the blood, fluid levels, pain, noise and a whole host of other factors.

SO HOW CAN ALL THIS AFFECT YOUR FAT LEVELS?

There are a number of theories about this, with both physiological and psychological changes thought to play a part. Mood certainly effects eating behaviours, with research showing that stress increases the tendency to eat high-sugar, high-fat foods (Torres, 2007). This desire may stem from the fact that eating these 'comfort' foods is associated with pleasure and in the short term decreases the stress levels within the body. The stress response is, however, varied, with some people opting for comfort foods and gaining weight, while others decrease food intake and lose weight in times of stress (Torres, 2007; Kivimaki et al, 2006).

Physiologically, stress may increase the risk of weight gain through a number of different mechanisms including:

- Changes in thyroid function
- Changes in liver function
- Worsened digestion
- Impact on numerous hormones
- Elevated blood sugars
- Adrenal fatigue and exhaustion

Many of the above can be linked back to changes caused by stress to:

- The HPA axis
- The autonomic nervous system

Drapeau et al (2003) noted that stress increases activation of the HPA axis, which in turn elevates levels of cortisol. The higher levels of cortisol seem to increase hunger and promote fat storage around the visceral organs. Interestingly they also

HPA axis

The hypothalamic-pituitary-adrenal or HPA axis is a feedback system linking the hypothalamus and pituitary gland in the brain, and the adrenal glands in the kidneys. Between them these three control the body's response to stress and influence energy expenditure, digestion, mood and the immune response.

The autonomic nervous system controls all of the 'automatic' processes that occur in the body without conscious thought, such as breathing, heartbeat, blood pressure, digestion and the dilation and constriction of blood vessels.

suggest that central obesity itself can be perceived as a stress by the body, causing further activation of the HPA axis and a vicious cycle in which stress causes obesity, which in turn causes stress and so on. Coupled with a person's desire for high-fat and high-sugar foods in times of stress, it is easy to see how this could lead to considerably higher levels of central body fat over time.

As well as obesity, an overactive HPA axis and autonomic nervous system is linked to high blood pressure, insulin resistance and type 2 diabetes, high cholesterol, and the other factors that together are commonly referred to as metabolic syndrome.

HAPPY HORMONES

Many hormones serve more than one purpose in the body and a number can affect both our physiology and our psychology. This includes the hormone melatonin. It is believed to play a role in weight regulation; possibly through its importance in bringing about quality sleep. As you've seen, poor sleep affects appetite and melatonin is crucial for a good night's kip. It is thought that it may assist in regulating blood glucose and, as such, weight gain. It also plays a part in elevating mood along with a number of other hormones and neurotransmitters.

THYROXINE

As its name suggests, thyroxine is a hormone produced by the thyroid gland, located in the neck. Together with triiodothyronine, they are known as the thyroid hormones and are responsible for increasing BMR and metabolising carbohydrates, fats and proteins.

Thyroid UK (2010) say that 2 per cent of the UK population, most commonly women in their 40s and 50s, suffer from hypothyroidism or underactive thyroid. This decreases the body's ability to raise BMR and increases the likelihood of weight gain. The major cause of this is iodine deficiency, sometimes from poor diet and lifestyle factors but also from genetic defects or medical conditions such as Hashimoto's disease, an autoimmune illness that attacks the thyroid gland, decreasing its ability to produce thyroid hormones. Increased intakes of fish or shellfish can help but some cases may require supplementation or even medication. There are a plethora of symptoms if somebody suffers from hypothyroidism, with weight gain, excessive tiredness, breathlessness, hair loss and poor skin amongst them. Instructors should signpost any client presenting with any of these symptoms to their GP.

OTHER STUFF

As you have seen there is a big interplay of hormones working inside the body to store fat, burn fat, increase calorie burn or store energy away for a later date. But it isn't just hormones that do this, other substances in the brain and the stomach play their part too. In the brain and central nervous system, neurotransmitters send signals from nerves to cells in the body.

One important neurotransmitter, serotonin, has a well-known mood boosting effect but it has also been shown to regulate appetite. Serotonin regulates appetite through signals created from eating meals. It can suppress some substances that drive hunger such as neuropeptide Y, which controls appetite by monitoring the fullness of fat cells and suppressing ghrelin.

Serotonin levels rise after eating carbohydrates, at which time they increase feelings of satisfaction and suppress appetite. Because of this, contrary to what many have said in recent years, it has been proposed that eating carbohydrates could be used as way of assisting weight loss. The idea is simple, according to Wurtman and Frusztajer (2009); eat carbohydrates, increase serotonin and decrease appetite. Some of their main suggestions include:

- Take care not to consume too many carbohydrates. Eating poor quality and large amounts of carbohydrates could lead to weight gain.
- Try eating a carbohydrate meal later in the day. This can help to suppress appetite in the evening when many tend to reach for sugary snacks. It may also help to improve sleep quality.
- Limit proteins and fats with the evening meal, opting instead for breakfasts and lunches that are higher in concentrations of these.

They do, however, caution that consuming the wrong type of carbohydrates, namely highly processed, refined sugars, can be linked with stress and depression. Low mood means low serotonin

– so the body reaches for foods that it knows will help raise a smile. The problem here is that if sugary foods are regularly consumed to get the daily 'happiness fix', weight gain occurs and insulin sensitivity decreases. In essence, the high-sugar lifestyle may become addictive – searching for a proper 'hit' – through the same mechanisms that lead to any substance abuse. So while carbohydrates can be helpful, the quality of the food consumed has a major impact.

Another neurotransmitter, dopamine, may also have a role to play. It also has links to mood and is involved in creating the smooth movement of muscles; Parkinson's disease is an autoimmune disease where dopamine-making cells in the brain are destroyed, impacting many of the body's functions, especially movement. It is also believed that dopamine plays a role in telling the brain that it is time to stop eating. Epstein et al (2007) studied 29 obese and 45 non-obese adults to discover if their dopamine levels had any impact on their appetite. Their results show that people with lower dopamine levels found food more rewarding and subsequently consumed more calories, possibly explaining a mechanism for their weight gain.

What about your genes? Is the reason for bigger jeans of the blue denim variety all down to genes of the deoxyribonucleic acid kind? Well, as we saw in the section on risk factors, hundreds of genes have been discovered that suggest an increased risk for some weight gain depending on their genetic code. Ravussin and Bogardus (2000) suggest that genetics may affect the respiratory quotient, a measure of the percentage of fat and carbohydrate a person burns when breathing. It may also impact food intake and metabolic rate, as well as influencing behaviours such as the desire to eat or the tendency to be sedentary.

What is clear though is that genes alone cannot cause obesity. They merely make someone more susceptible, and major lifestyle factors like exercise and diet then influence weight gain more significantly. This is evidenced by the speed at which obesity levels have risen across the world. It takes thousands of years for changes in genes to occur, yet in 30 years levels of obesity have grown out of all proportion. The Centers for Disease Control and Prevention (2013) in a review of genetics and obesity refer to the 'thrifty genotype hypothesis'; this argument notes that the human body is in many ways designed to survive in times of famine by storing fat efficiently, but that in modern society where food is readily available this may be working against us, leading to expanding waistlines.

SUMMARY

- Metabolism consists of anabolism and catabolism. There are various calculations for estimating Basal Metabolic Rate and total daily energy requirements.
- Numerous hormones have a role to play in weight management and levels of these are influenced by lifestyle behaviours.
- Neurotransmitters may also play their part in affecting hunger and satiety, and indirectly affect food intake through changes in mood.

MEASURING UP – CONSULTATIONS WITH CLIENTS AND FITNESS TESTING

// **3**

Before someone begins their weight loss journey, it is important to carry out some sort of review of what he or she wants and their current health status. There are a number of things you'll need to consider here. Are you, or is your client, ready to begin an exercise programme without seeing their GP first? What are their goals? Where are they starting from? What have they done in the past and did it work? This section helps you to work with your client to discover the answers to these questions, and more.

Rapport

The Merriam-Webster Online Dictionary (2013) says that the word rapport derives from an old French word meaning 'to bring back'. This is a nice link to the modern day meaning of the word, as it is to do with how well you get on with another person and if the relationship is reciprocated.

In recent years you may have seen information about using 'mirroring techniques' (copying someone's body language, essentially reflecting their actions back to them) to build rapport. In my experience these can help if used appropriately, if done blatantly the other person just thinks you are strange. In fact it is not only body language that can be mirrored, words used, pace and volume of voice can be reflected back, as can everything from breathing rate to blinking. While these can create an environment for rapport to be built, rapport itself goes much deeper than this. It is about finding similarities, respecting differences and having trust in, and feeling comfortable around others.

You may have noticed that with people who you are close to you seem to use the same words or sit in the same way without thinking about it. This is because you have such a deep level of rapport. With clients you need to build enough rapport in the early stages to earn their trust. Without this they'll be unlikely to want to reveal the sensitive information you need in order to create a programme that suits their needs. Many overweight and obese clients may also be new to exercise or to a gym and, as such, having someone they feel comfortable with is going to make it far more likely that they will stick to their new, healthier lifestyle.

CONSULTATIONS WITH CLIENTS

Why do this? If you're going to create an exercise and lifestyle programme for someone who wants to lose weight there is a lot of information you'll need to gather in order to be able to do it effectively. However, even before you gather any information, you need to develop a good level of rapport with your client and get to know a bit more about what makes them tick.

WHY, WHEN, WHERE AND HOW?

Why carry out fitness assessments and health screens with your clients? There are a host of benefits for testing, but also some possible drawbacks. The table below provides a useful summary.

It is best to be open and up front with clients from the outset, explaining the purpose of, benefits and drawbacks of assessments and giving them the option to choose which, if any, are carried out. It may be essential to carry out certain assessments like blood pressure to ensure that clients are safe to exercise but others can be open to personal choice. Obviously, being able to show results is important and explaining the benefits and how you will carry tests out can often allay any fears from clients, but if a client has strong objections and it risks the likelihood of them not continuing their programme then they may need to be left out. Tests can always be done further down the line as a client's confidence and self-esteem increases.

Table 3.1	Benefits and drawbacks of fitness assessments
Benefits and drawbacks	**Key points**
Benefits of fitness testing	• Allows people to track progress towards goals • Provides motivation through recognising success • Shows changes that occur in body composition when weight may not have changed • Shows that changes are not taking place and that adaptations to the programme or to lifestyle need to be made • Identifies any possible reasons for referral to a medical professional if required
Drawbacks of fitness testing	• Some people may be anxious about having fitness assessments, especially those that require measurement of their size or shape • Some tests can entail physical contact or removal of clothing, which may be uncomfortable for many, especially if they have only recently met you • Some may become demotivated by seeing poor results so it is important to frame them in the correct context, especially the first measurement

WHEN SHOULD YOU TEST?

This depends very much on the individual. It is extremely useful to test before any exercise and lifestyle changes are made to enable you to see the progress being made, what works and what doesn't. The frequency of tests after that depends very much on the person you are working with. Some may prefer to be weighed regularly to ensure they are on track and so a weekly weigh-in may be preferable. Weight loss in this time will, however, be small and may not be motivational so it may be best to opt for fortnightly or monthly weigh-ins for those who are motivated by seeing bigger results. Daily weighing should be discouraged, as there are many variables that may change it such as hydration, food in the stomach, etc.

For other tests such as body fat percentage and circumference measurements, monthly measurement may be the best option. Any less and the results gained may not be enough to motivate the client, any more and they may lose their way as they can't see any tangible changes for their efforts. Tests of physical fitness also require a reasonable amount of time between them to enable changes to occur. This may be more frequent for those new to exercise, as they will see progress quicker than experienced exercisers. Monthly fitness tests to fit in line with other tests may be appropriate.

As well as physical fitness, you may also wish to measure the functional ability of clients, looking at their ability to perform everyday tasks. This may be especially relevant where a client has limitations to movement caused by being overweight.

WHAT ABOUT THE TIME OF DAY?

This can make a big difference to test results. Height is a good example, with people being taller first thing in the morning than they are later in the day (the spine compacts down as the day progresses due to the effects of our body weight passing through the discs). Weight can also be affected due to food in the stomach and hydration levels, as can performance in physical tests. The body is also subject to circadian rhythms where body temperature, blood pressure, muscle strength and a host of other physiological factors change across the course of 24 hours. For guidance on the best times of day to carry out assessments refer to the information on each of the individual tests that follow later in this section. Time of the month may also be a factor to consider for women entering their menstrual cycle as this may affect results, especially in weight and waist circumference tests. Repeatability is key – so whichever times of day and month are used in the initial tests should be repeated throughout.

WHERE SHOULD YOU CARRY OUT TESTS?

You need to consider issues such as comfort, privacy and safety. Taking personal measurements like weight, body fat and circumference measurements may be best done in a place that offers a degree of privacy, but at the same time working one on one with someone away from others can carry risks, both for safety and for accusations of poor practice. It can be difficult to defend against these if the only people present are the instructor and the client, so it can be wise to offer clients the opportunity to have a friend or family member come along if they wish. This can offer comfort for the client, protection against accusations of malpractice and an opportunity to ensure you have contact with an important member of your client's support crew who can help motivate and assist them to reach their goals.

Meeting new clients at their home may not always be preferable. While most people are genuine about their desire for support, instructors should not take unnecessary risks and it may be best to advise meeting at a neutral venue in the first instance. For those not working in a professional fitness facility it may be best to have a place you can rent for these sessions where other people are around and there is a professional atmosphere that allows for privacy where required.

HOW DO YOU MEASURE OVERWEIGHT/OBESITY LEVELS?

Depending on the tests chosen there are a number of different ways to measure weight and fat changes over time. These include Body Mass Index, body fat percentage, circumference measurements or even physiological changes linked to weight, such as blood glucose. Appropriate training and insurance is needed for the latter.

HEALTH SCREENING

Before taking any physical measurements be sure to carry out some form of health screening. With clients this may involve completion of a Physical Activity Readiness Questionnaire (PAR-Q), Health Commitment Statement (HCS) or suitable alternative health questionnaire.

It is also strongly advised that you take a blood pressure reading, because being overweight is a risk factor for hypertension and heart disease. As hypertension will likely have no symptoms, measurement is a good idea. You can use an automatic blood pressure machine to do this. Ensure the client is rested and at ease and has not drunk caffeine or alcohol before the test. You may wish to perform more than one reading dependent on

the initial score. High blood pressure is defined as 140/90 mmHg so if either reading is above these scores repeat a second time. You can do a third reading after a few minutes if still high. If at this point the readings are still elevated then you should send the client to their GP for further checks. Be sure to explain why you are doing this and remain calm while emphasising that it is important to have the checks in order not to cause any unnecessary distress. *Do not diagnose* based on the readings you have taken. All you can say is that the readings you took on the day were higher than they should be and that a medical practitioner would need to follow this up before the client can begin exercising.

Some may work in an environment where it is possible to carry out finger-prick blood glucose or cholesterol testing. As the risk of heart disease and diabetes is elevated with increased weight, these can be useful tests and should be referred to a medical practitioner if the results gained are outside of the norms. Clients should have fasted for eight hours prior to having these tests done to ensure they are reliable so early morning testing is often best as it is easier to go without food overnight. A reading of greater than 5 mmol/l for cholesterol and of greater than 7 mmol/l for glucose should prompt a visit to their GP.

BODY MASS INDEX (BMI)

This is calculated by dividing your weight in kilograms by your height squared. It gives an indication of overall size and in many people a high BMI can be a sign of elevated fat levels leading to increased risk of numerous illnesses. Originally known as the Quetelet Index after Adolphe Quetelet, a Belgian mathematician, astronomer and statistician, it

Table 3.2 A simple BMI classification tool

Benefits	Drawbacks
• Quick and easy to carry out • Relatively cheap in terms of equipment required • Fairly well understood and recognised by clients	• Doesn't take into account muscle mass • Doesn't tell you where body fat sits • Too simplistic on its own to provide any conclusive information • The tables generally used don't distinguish between age, race and gender

was designed in the mid-nineteenth century to compare the size of populations in what he termed 'social studies', revealing when in life people tended to grow. In the third quarter of the twentieth century this little-known measurement began to gain notoriety in the medical world, being associated in a series of studies with an increased risk of disease and mortality. From this point onwards it grew in popularity and became a common way of measuring obesity and risk of illness in the medical world, but in recent years the usefulness of this measure has been questioned.

It is now recognised that it is not purely size that indicates risk for heart disease and other illness, but how much of the body is fat and where that fat sits, as well as a host of other things going on internally. Some people who have a high BMI have low body fat levels and high muscle mass. Rugby players and American footballers are often good examples of this so their risk for disease is not necessarily elevated.

The World Health Organization (WHO) provides a useful classification of BMI (see Table 3.3).

Table 3.3 BMI Norms table

Classification	BMI (kg/m^2)
Underweight	Less than 18.5
Severe thinness	Less than 16
Moderate thinness	16–16.99
Mild thinness	17–18.49
Normal weight	18.5–24.9
Overweight	25–29.9
Obese	More than 30
Obese class I	30–34.9
Obese class II	35–39.9
Obese class III	More than 40

(adapted from the WHO International Classification of adult underweight, overweight and obesity according to BMI)

Even these classifications have been the point of much debate, with many arguing that they should be specific to different ethnicities. In 2002, the WHO reviewed BMI classifications because research suggested Asian populations should have lower cut-off points due to their tendency towards smaller frame-sizes. Because of disparity between different populations in Asia and a lack of consensus, they decided to keep BMI classifications the same for all at present. Since then, however, some Asian countries have set their own classifications of overweight and obese according to BMI. The Harvard School of Public Health have summarised these and they are presented in Table 3.4:

Table 3.4	Region specific BMI classifications	
Country	BMI classification for overweight	BMI classification for obesity
China/Japan	24 (kg/m^2)	28 (kg/m^2)
India	23 (kg/m^2)	27 (kg/m^2)

There are also different measurement protocols for children developed by both the WHO and the National Health Service in the UK. The NHS website has a useful tool to calculate children's BMIs. This converts the BMI result for a child into a 'centile score', showing how they compare to other children of the same age and gender and identifying which category they then fall into, such as normal weight or overweight. (See www.nhs.uk/tools/pages/healthyweight calculator.aspx)

MEASURING BMI

To measure BMI you will need the following equipment:

- A height scale. Preferably use one that is clinically accurate such as a stadiometer (has a footplate to stand on and a moving arm that rests on the head when measured, see Figure 3.1).
- Weighing scales.

To measure height, ensure the scale is a placed on a flat, level surface. The person should remove their shoes and stand on the footplate, heels against the base of the scale. They should stand tall but relaxed with their bottom, upper back and back of their head resting against the scale with the normal curves in their spine maintained. The head should face forwards with the eyes approximately level with the top of the ears. The moving arm should be pulled down to the top of the head, flattening any hair in the way and the reading taken while the person is still on the scale. Look for heels lifting off the floor or the head tilting up, which will both push the arm higher and decrease the accuracy of the reading.

The time of day at which height is measured is important. People are generally tallest immediately after waking, most likely because the intervertebral discs, which are composed largely of water, have expanded. During the day when we are mostly upright, they compress making us shorter. Many studies have shown a decrease in height of around 1.5–3 cm across the course of a day (Krishan and Vij, 2007), although some show smaller decreases. The key is to keep measurement time consistent to ensure repeatability and decrease risks for error, but if the statistics are

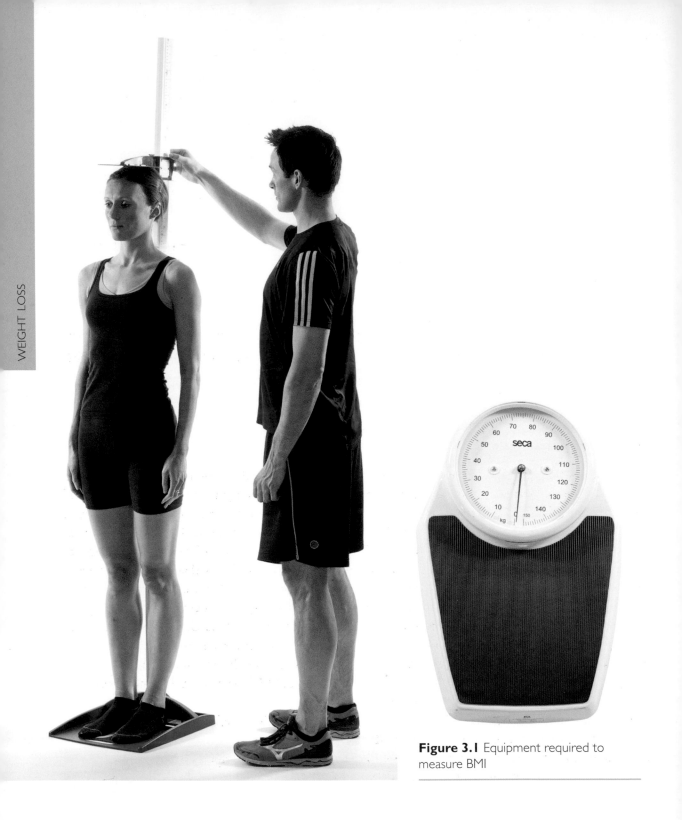

Figure 3.1 Equipment required to measure BMI

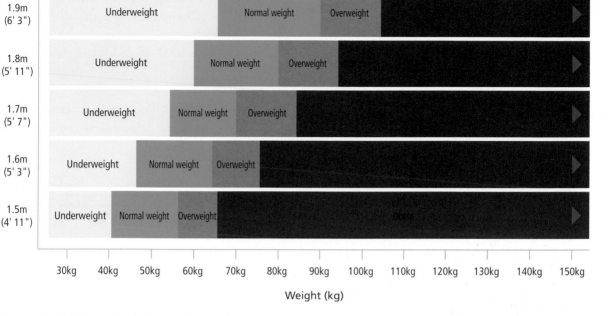

Figure 3.2 A simple BMI classification tool

anything to go by, people will probably want to be measured first thing in the morning as they will be taller and their BMI scores lower.

Weighing also requires a strict protocol to ensure accuracy. Scales should be calibrated if possible (some come with set weights to do this while others may need to be sent away), or at least the same set of scales used each time to minimise variation. Place the scales on a flat, even surface and ensure the dial is set to zero before the client steps on. Ensure the person being weighed is wearing light clothing, has removed their shoes, watch and any items such as wallet, coins or mobile phone from their pockets. When they are on the scales, ensure that the client stands tall with weight evenly through both feet and is not holding on to anything for support or leaning against a wall as

this will decrease the accuracy of the measurement. For consistency, weigh at the same time of day, and for women consider the impact of the menstrual cycle. The latter can be challenging as it involves tactfully asking a personal question. It is best to be clear as to the things that can impact weight as this gives your client a reason as to why you are asking. As always, give them the opportunity not to answer if they'd rather. Consistency of methodology is important for identifying progress.

Once you have a height and weight reading you can work out BMI using the following calculation:

$$\text{Weight (kg)} \div \text{Height}^2 \text{ (m)}$$

Let's look at an example.

Clinton weights 83 kg and is 180 cm tall.

1. Calculate the square of Clinton's height. Convert his height into metres, (as this is the measurement for the calculation) then multiply it by itself. Do not round it up or down at this stage to ensure accuracy.

$$1.8 \times 1.8 = 3.24$$

2. Divide Clinton's weight by his height squared. You can round to a whole number once you have this score

$$83 \div 3.24 = 25.6 \ (26)$$

Use the BMI table on page 28 to work out his classification. Alternatively, use the diagram on page 31 instead.

Clinton has a BMI of 26 and is classified as overweight.

Although very useful, because of its limitations, BMI should be done alongside the subsequent tests where possible.

WAIST CIRCUMFERENCE AND WAIST-TO-HIPS RATIO

In recent times there has been growing evidence that waist measurement might provide a useful alternative or supplement to BMI. This is

The long and short of it

While height and weight are fairly simple to measure, they can be extremely sensitive subjects so care is needed when measuring. Follow the tips below to ensure that people feel comfortable being measured:

- Explain the benefits and drawbacks of the tests and of BMI, especially in showing progress over time, regardless of their starting point.
- Offer the choice to opt out of the tests if they wish.
- Talk them through the protocols and explain what you are doing at every stage.
- Discuss issues such as personal space, finding out their preferences.
- Ask how the client prefers to see the measurements; would they like readings in centimetres or feet and inches? Would they like weight measurements in kilograms or stones and pounds? Carry a weight conversion chart with you to make this a quick, easy process. Some may prefer not to see the readings at all initially, but be willing to do them in order that they can see their progress later on.
- Ask the person what they expect their results to be; this helps set expectations and you can judge how to feedback readings.
- Talk around the topics beforehand to gather an idea of how sensitive people are towards the readings. Consider this when phrasing feedback about results.
- Consider your body language, tone of voice and use of words when carrying out the assessments.
- Ensure the person is comfortable in the environment in which the assessments take place.

Table 3.5	Table of norms for waist circumference	
	Increased risk of illness	**High risk of illness**
Men	94–101 cm (37–39 in)	102 cm (40 in)+ 90 cm (35 in)+ for Asian men
Women	80–87 cm (32–34 in)	88 cm (34.5 in)+ 80 cm (32 in)+ for Asian women

adapted from data from the NHS Choices (2012) and the International Diabetes Foundation (2007)

because it is a marker of visceral fat, the stuff that deposits in and around the vital organs, decreasing their ability to work properly and increasing the likelihood of illness occurring, especially diabetes and heart disease.

Some people carry more fat around their hips, in particular women, and are referred to as *gynoid* or 'pear-shaped'. The risk for heart disease in this shape is thought to be lower than in people who are *android* or 'apple-shaped' and carry their body fat around their middle, although some recent research questions this, showing that fat stored around the buttocks may secrete abnormal levels of chemerin, a protein that can increase inflammation in the body (Golden, 2013). Up to now it has also been generally accepted that the apple-shape is more common in men, which has been linked to the higher rate of heart attacks in men. However, central obesity is becoming more common in women, as is the number of cardiovascular events (Towfighi et al, 2009).

Waist measurements are simple, quick and easy to take, requiring only a tape measure, which is cheap to buy. It is also a method of measuring that people can understand and relate to, as many desire to decrease size in order to fit into clothes. On the flipside, waist measurements do have some drawbacks: if done poorly they can feel invasive; cheap tape measures may stretch; and if taken in the wrong place measurements can be inaccurate. Some will naturally have broader waists due to frame size or higher muscle mass, although the general consensus is that waist measurements provide a useful, reliable indication of risk.

CARRYING OUT WAIST CIRCUMFERENCE MEASUREMENTS

Use the following guidelines to carry out effective waist measurements with clients:

- Use a non-stretch tape measure. Some have metal clasps at the end that you can loop the tape measure into, minimising personal contact when carrying out tests.
- Make sure you have a tape measure long enough for more overweight or obese clients. Failure to do so can really lower self-esteem making it less likely they will continue.
- Refrain from the 'big hug' approach. Instead of pressing your body against someone, ask them to take the tape measure and pass it around themselves.

- Those being measured should wear light clothing to prevent errors in readings. After handing the client the tape to pass round, put it into the metal clasp if available and draw tight to the skin at the height of the navel (belly button). If clients are obese, the navel may have dropped as the stomach hangs forwards. Instead use a determined point to measure such as a bony landmark. Record this and use the same point next time for consistency. Take the measurement in centimetres but offer the reading to the client in inches if they prefer, you can record both. When taking the readings stand to the side of the client. Standing or kneeling in front or behind the client can be intimidating and invade personal space.

Use the following World Health Organization (2008) guidelines for measurement:

- Clients should stand tall, arms by their sides with their feet close together.
- Clients should breathe normally and measurements should be taken at the end of exhalation.
- Abdominals should be relaxed and ideally the measurement should be taken in the morning before eating or drinking.
- The tape measure should be tight to the skin but not constricting.
- Some tape measures have coloured markings to identify the waist circumference classification. Alternatively, use the table on page 33.
- Some may have a very different notion of where their waist is as clothing 'waistlines' tend to sit lower, so it is important to explain the protocol and the reasons for it.
- Provide the client with the readings and the classification, feeding back honestly but sensitively.

A commonly used similar test is the waist-to-hips ratio. This uses the following simple formula to calculate future risk for cardiovascular disease, diabetes and related illnesses.

$$\text{Waist circumference (cm)} \div \text{hip circumference (cm)}$$

Take the waist measurement in the same way as described above. Hips should be read as the widest visible circumference as recommended by

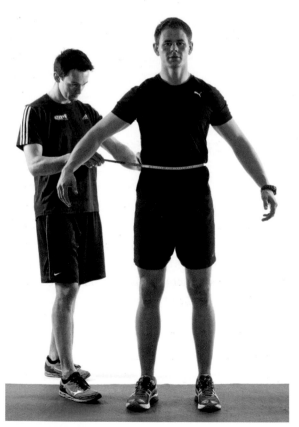

Figure 3.3 Measuring the circumference of the waist

the World Health Organization (2008) and it is advisable to take three readings in the area to ensure you find this measure. Look for the widest point and as before ask the client to pass the tape measure around. Attach into the clasp if available and measure off on the side. Ensure the tape measure is not twisted and is parallel to the floor. Once you've recorded your measurement, move the tape measure up two centimetres and take another, then down two centimetres below the original reading. You should take the widest of the three readings or an average.

Now you have a waist and hips measurement it's time to do the Carol Vorderman bit. Feel free to use a calculator though.

Alice is 62 years old and had the following readings:

Waist – 77 cm
Hips – 94 cm
77 ÷ 94 = 0.82

The NHS (2013) considers a waist-to-hips ratio of above 1.0 in men and above 0.85 in women to represent an increased risk of heart disease and diabetes. Bray and Gray (1988) developed more detailed categories for waist-to-hip ratio readings that are easily located on the Internet, just type in 'waist-to-hip ratio chart' and look in Google images for examples. In reference to Alice above, she is just below the NHS cut-off point of 0.85 for women and, as such, has moderately increased risk of coronary heart disease and type 2 diabetes.

The big question is whether to only do waist circumference, just waist-to-hips ratio, or both? Both are validated tests and act as useful indicators of health status. Also, both can show changes as someone loses weight and therefore act as markers of progress. Because of the challenge of obtaining consistently accurate hip measurements, waist circumference may be the better option. Waist-to-hips ratio scores can sometimes be a little misleading in people with certain body shapes. Those carrying a lot of fat around the hips may come out with a low score but as you've seen already, fat around the buttocks may pose a bigger risk than was once thought. Ectomorphs who could be described as 'straight up, straight down' may have completely normal BMI, waist circumference and body fat readings but may show as higher risk on the waist-to-hip ratio because the two readings are closer due to their often narrower hips.

The best advice is to take both readings alongside BMI and body fat percentage. Having a 360-degree view of all of the measurements empowers you with a wealth of information, allowing suitable advice to be given.

OTHER CIRCUMFERENCE MEASUREMENTS

You or your client may not just want to know about waist or hip measurements, what about the rest of the body, such as arms or legs? Well, although there are no clinical norms for these to compare against and you can't identify long-term risk for illness, there's a lot to be gained from these measurements.

- They're very useful for showing shape change over time and take into account the fact that some people lose weight from different areas at differing rates.
- They link closely to personal goals; some may want more toned 'bingo wings' or for their legs to look better in shorts.

- They give numbers that can be used to set SMART goals and quantify progress.
- You can read them in centimetres or inches depending on the individual's preference.

The key for the measurements is a consistent method. As long as you use the same protocol each time you can ensure that what you're measuring is a valid marker of change. Below are some suggestions for how to do this:

ARMS

- Welcome to the gun show. An easy way to measure arms consistently is to ask the individual to raise their arm to the side and tense their biceps.
- Readings can be taken around the widest point visible.
- Move the tape measure slightly and repeat measurement to ensure the widest circumference is found.

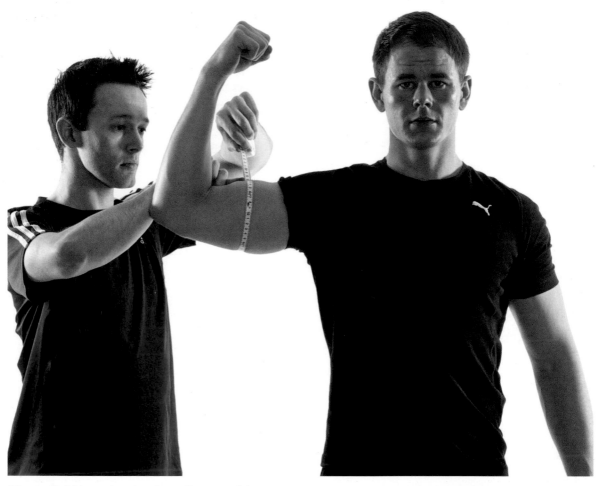

Figure 3.4 Measuring the circumference of the arm

LEGS (UPPER)

- Ask the individual to step forwards with one leg, keeping the weight on the back foot.
- They should place their arms by their sides, fingers outstretched.
- Ensure they are standing tall and not reaching down the leg.
- Place the tape measure under the tip of the index finger, to hold it as you wrap it around the leg.
- Ensure the tape measure is parallel to the floor and not twisted.

LEGS (LOWER)

- Estimate the widest point of the calf visually.
- The individual should stand tall and the calf muscle should be relaxed.
- Once measured, move the tape measure up two centimetres and repeat.
- Do this again two centimetres below the original reading and take the widest of the three measurements.
- Alternatively you can measure a set distance up from the malleolus (bony bit on the outside of the ankle). This would ensure a consistent reading each time.

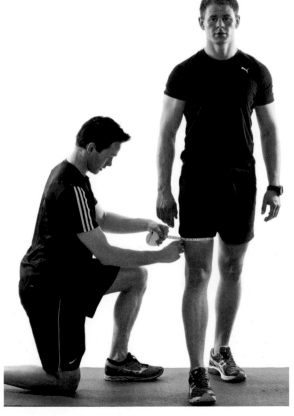

Figure 3.5 Measuring the circumference of the upper leg

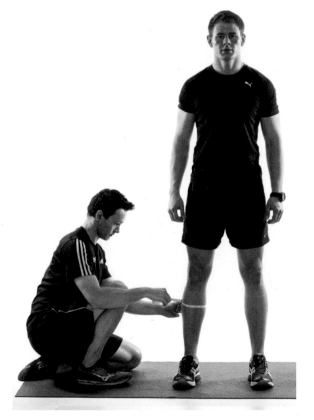

Figure 3.6 Measuring the circumference of the lower leg

BODY FAT PERCENTAGE

Important to clients as a measure of their progress, and to fitness and health professionals, body fat percentage is arguably one of the strongest indicators of health. However, at this stage there is minimal research on the link between lean mass and fat mass on disease risk, with most of the focus on BMI or waist circumference. Some research has identified important links between lean mass and diabetes, cardiovascular disease and ageing (Ferreira et al, 2004; Castaneda et al, 2002; Wolfe, 2006).

Physical problems can also occur if body fat is too low, especially in women where fat plays an essential role in menstrual function and hormone production. Men can in theory have as little as

What is body fat?

There are two types of fat in the body:

- Essential fat – as its name suggests this fat is very much needed to help the body function. It includes fat found in muscle tissue, the brain and other organs, bone marrow and nerves. In the latter, for example, it helps to make the myelin sheath that surrounds nerves, accounting for around 80 per cent of its total mass and allowing electrical impulses to be passed effectively around the body.
- Storage fat – this is the fat that sits beneath your skin (known as subcutaneous fat) and around your organs (visceral fat). Some is needed to protect internal organs and keep the body warm, with the rest stored as energy reserves. However, many people store too much these days due to a combination of overeating and sedentary lifestyles.

Fats as a whole are known as *lipids*, originating from the ancient Greek word 'lipos', meaning fat. When foods are consumed they contain a mixture of fatty acids, some saturated, some unsaturated and some trans-fatty acids. These will be discussed in more detail in Chapter 5. When stored they are converted to triacylglycerol, or *triglycerides* as they are more commonly referred to. Triglycerides consist of three fatty acids and a glycerol atom and are stored within fat cells known as *adipocytes*.

Fat storage occurs when levels of fatty acids are high in the blood, such as after a meal. Insulin is released from the pancreas in response to this, and fatty acids are drawn into the adipocytes to be stored for later use. Should levels of fatty acids in the blood drop, for example if someone has not eaten for a while, adipocytes will release fats into the bloodstream as fatty acids in order to provide a ready supply of energy. This can also occur during exercise when energy is required to power movement.

During childhood, levels of body fat can increase through growth in the size of adipocytes and an increase in the number of fat cells. As adults, little change occurs in the number of fat cells, with cell numbers increasing only in extreme obesity when the current adipocytes are full to the brim. Otherwise, adults maintain a consistent level of around 75 billion adipocytes. (McArdle et al, 2010, p.800).

3 per cent body fat, while the leanest women may have around 12 per cent, although some argue that 17–22 per cent is needed for menstrual functioning (McArdle et al, 2010, p. 737).

Studies also show that body fat percentage can be high, even in those with normal BMIs and waist circumferences, and as such it is an important measure as it may be less apparent than the more visual tests (Deurenberg-Yap and Chew, 2002). Clients often talk about how they look in the mirror, how they feel in their clothes and what they would like to tone up. All of these things are not about weight loss; they are about fat loss while maintaining lean muscle tissue.

It's clear that body fat is an important marker of health, so let's look at how it can be measured. There are various methods, some of them simple and doable in a gym environment, others more scientific and requiring far more expensive equipment and time to carry out. These include:

- Bioelectrical impedance analysis (BIA)
- Skinfold measurements
- Hydrostatic weighing
- Bod Pod
- Magnetic resonance imaging (MRI)

BIOELECTRICAL IMPEDANCE ANALYSIS (BIA)

BIA has become reasonably commonplace in recent years, with many companies selling scales or handheld devices to the public. It works by sending a small electrical current between electrodes. On scales these electrodes are placed within footplates for the individual to stand on, or in handheld devices the person grips two handles attached to the device. Some BIA scales have both a footplate and a handheld device, and other devices require special tabs such as those used for ECGs to be placed on the hand and foot with clips attaching these to the reading device.

How does it work? The measuring device sends an alternating current between the two electrodes. If you're worried about electrocuting someone just to test his or her body fat, then don't be, the current is small and cannot be felt. Water and lean

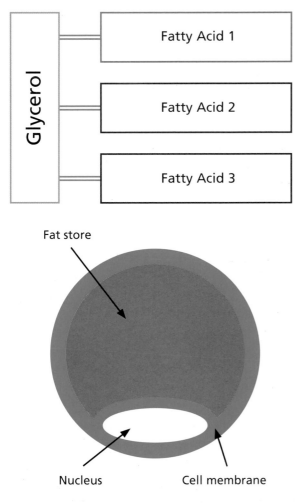

Figure 3.7 Fats: the basic structure of a triglyceride (top) and an adipoctye (bottom)

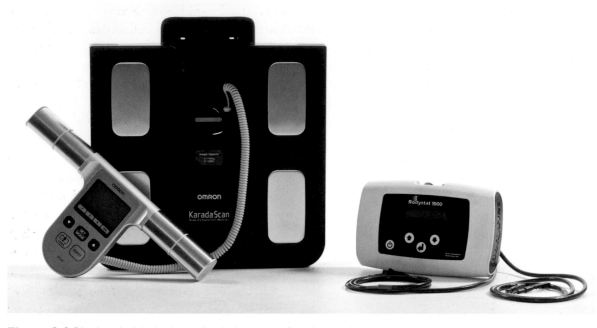

Figure 3.8 Bioelectrical Impedance Analysis: types of testing equipment

mass conduct electrical current better than fat and bone. This is because they contain more electrolytes. By calculating the resistance (or impedance) of the water to the flow of the current, the machines can estimate lean mass and body fat percentage.

The machines used are programmed with calculations based on age, gender, height, etc. and these are inputted before carrying out the test. The BIA scale can then estimate body fat based on this information and the resistance to flow measured.

SKINFOLD MEASUREMENT

Alongside BIA, skinfolds are one of the most commonly used methods for estimating body fat percentage in individuals, the former probably more common these days due to the fact that it is quicker and less invasive. As their name suggests,

skinfolds involve the pinching of the skin to get measurements that can then be used to predict body fat levels based on gender and age. This is because, as you have seen, much of a person's fat stores lie subcutaneously and so equations have been created that predict total fat levels for a given series of measurements.

There are a various testing methodologies, using different measurement areas, or 'sites' around the body, some using three, some four, seven or even nine. In theory, if done correctly, the more sites used the more accurate the results gained will be. However, more sites take a lot more time to measure and increase the risk of inaccuracy. Calipers are used to measure each site. These are in essence a big pair of tweezers, consisting of a handle for the tester to hold, a trigger that allows them to pull open the caliper and a dial that provides a reading in millimetres. The tester identifies the site and marks it to ensure accuracy, pulls the skin away from the body ensuring that they are only taking fat and not muscle and while holding it, places the calipers around the site, releases the trigger so that they sit flush to the skin and then takes the reading after two seconds.

It takes a lot of practice to become skilled in using calipers and, if inaccurate, readings can vary greatly and are of little use. It can also be uncomfortable, even painful for the client if carried out incorrectly. If done well, however, skinfold measurement is a valid test of body fat and can be almost as accurate as hydrostatic weighing (Oppliger et al, 1987). This is discussed in more detail on page 51. Accuracy depends not only on the skill of the measurer but also on the tools used. Some calipers available at lower costs measure only in two-millimetre increments and may not

be accurately calibrated leading to innacuarcy, whereas more precise models such as Harpenden calipers record in 0.2-millimetre increments and have the springs calibrated for accuracy. Even these need occasional recalibration to ensure they remain accurate. They can be sent back to the manufacturer for this procedure.

One of the major considerations with calipers is invasiveness. Carrying out the tests requires a fair bit of physical contact and if someone is not comfortable with you in their personal space then it may be best to sacrifice the accuracy gained in favour of ensuring they feel comfortable. High quality testing would need the client to wear minimal clothing, or even to remove some clothes to ensure you can get the skinfold reading from exactly the right place. It is wise to discuss this with your client, explain the process and the benefits and to let them decide if they wish to have it done.

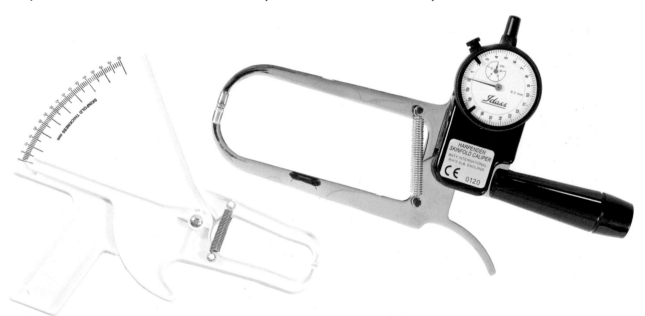

Figure 3.9 Pinch an inch: calipers for body fat testing

The table below identifies the caliper measurement sites that are commonly used in the different measurement protocols for both men and women. There are many different combinations in use though.

Let's have a look at how to carry out these measurements. There are some guidelines that apply to every measurement you take, regardless of the protocol used. Unless there is a good reason, always take measurements from the right side of the body. This is the side used in the scientific studies from which the norms are taken to ensure consistency between all tests. Take the pinches of the skin with the thumb and forefinger of your left hand and ensure you place calipers at right angles to the pinch, around two centimetres away from the fingers. The caliper should be placed halfway between the base and the top of the fold and take the finger completely off the trigger. Do this slowly to prevent the calipers from snapping on to the skin, which can be painful. Wait two seconds before taking the reading and then repeat a second time to ensure accuracy. If the measurements are not the same then you should take a third. Depending on protocols, you can then take the average of the closest two, or choose the median (middle number) of the three (ExRx.net, 2013). Finally, make sure you can gain

Table 3.6	Caliper measurement sites				
	3–site	4–site (version 1)	4–site (version 2)	7–site	9–site
Biceps (front of upper arm)		✓			✓
Triceps (back of upper arm)	✓ (female)	✓	✓	✓	✓
Pectoral (chest)	✓ (male)	✓		✓	✓
Subscapular (below the shoulder blade)		✓		✓	✓
Abdomen (stomach)	✓ (male)		✓	✓	✓
Suprailiac (above the pelvis)	✓ (female)		✓	✓	✓
Midaxillary (below the armpit)				✓	✓
Thigh (front or sometimes back of upper leg)	✓ (male and female)		✓	✓	✓
Gastrocnemius (back of the lower leg)					✓

proper access to the skinfold. Do not work around clothes and ensure the skin is not slippery, as this will decrease accuracy. This may be the case if the person is wearing moisturiser or suntan lotion, or if they are sweaty. If so, ask them to shower and dry off or postpone the test.

BICEPS

Have the client rest their arm by their side, palm up. Find the midpoint (the belly) of the biceps muscle, at the very front, halfway between the elbow joint and the bony point of the acromion process at the shoulder. The reading will likely be at around the height of the nipple. For accuracy, measure between the two points using a tape measure. Draw a horizontal line using something that will wash off, an eyebrow pencil is good. Make a cross by drawing down through the centre of the muscle and then pinch the skin one to two centimetres above the cross. Take the caliper reading on the cross as described above.

TRICEPS

Flex the arm and use a tape measure to mark the midpoint between the acromion process (bony bit at the back of the shoulder) and the olecranon process (elbow). Draw a horizontal line and then complete the cross marking through the belly of the muscle. Take the pinch vertically one to two centimetres above the cross and take the reading on the cross. This will be slightly higher up than the biceps reading.

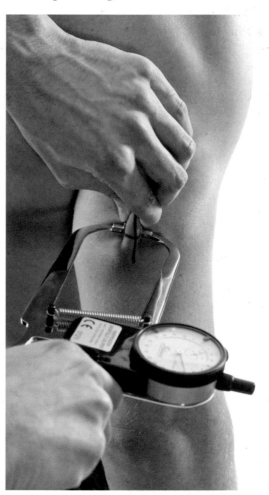

Figure 3.11 Tricep measurement

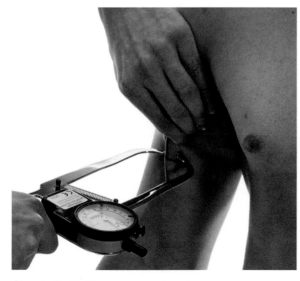

Figure 3.10 Bicep measurement

PECTORAL (CHEST)

Measure halfway between the anterior axiallary fold (the crease at the armpit) and the nipple. For men the reading is taken halfway between the two, for women one third of the way. This can be a very personal and invasive test so be careful where you put your hands. You can ask people to hold the tape measure at the nipple or you can estimate the measure visually; doing so will decrease the accuracy of the reading but client comfort is paramount. Draw the mark on the diagonal at 45 degrees and make a cross to take the reading as with other measurements.

SUBSCAPULAR (BELOW THE SHOULDER BLADE)

Find the inferior angle (lowest point) of the scapula bone. In some people you may struggle to find this so you can make it easier by asking them to place their arm behind their back as if in an arm lock. Obviously don't turn it into a wrestling move. This should raise the scapula

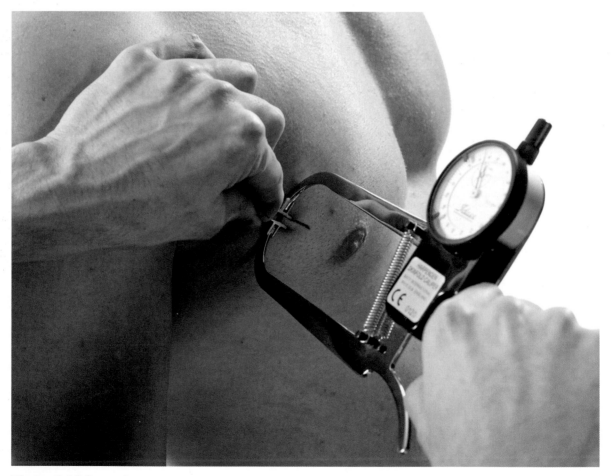

Figure 3.12 Pectoral measurement

making the point easier to locate. Measure two centimetres directly below and mark a line at 45 degrees down away from the midline of the body. Take the measure along this line.

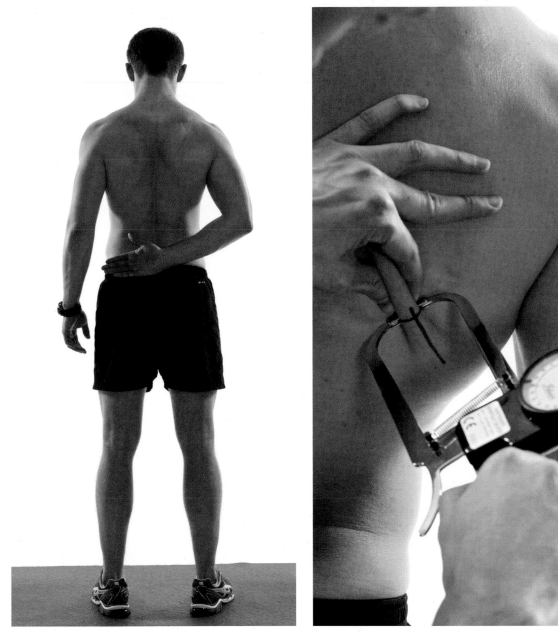

Figure 3.13 Subscapular measurement

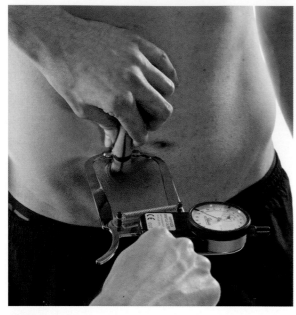

Figure 3.14 Abdomen measurement

ABDOMEN

Make a mark five centimetres to the right of the belly button (navel). Draw a vertical line and take the pinch along the line at the height of the belly button.

SUPRAILIAC (ABOVE THE PELVIS)

Find the iliac crest on the top of the pelvis. To do this, stand to the right-hand side, place your fingertips onto where you think the crest is located and ask the client to perform a side bend (laterally flex) towards you. If your fingertips disappear they're likely too high as the pelvis won't be moving. You should be able now to find the top of the bone. Draw a horizontal line immediately above the crest. The measure can be taken horizontally here, or some protocols will suggest also locating the anterior portion of the iliac crest,

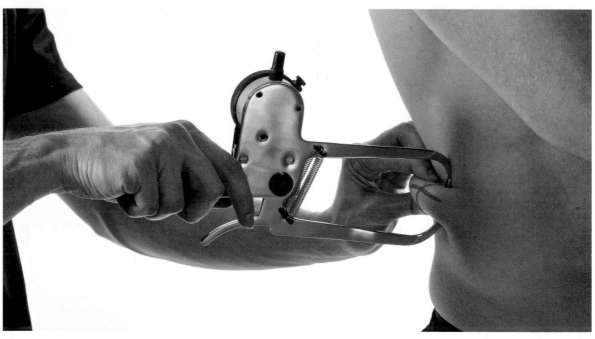

Figure 3.15 Suprailiac

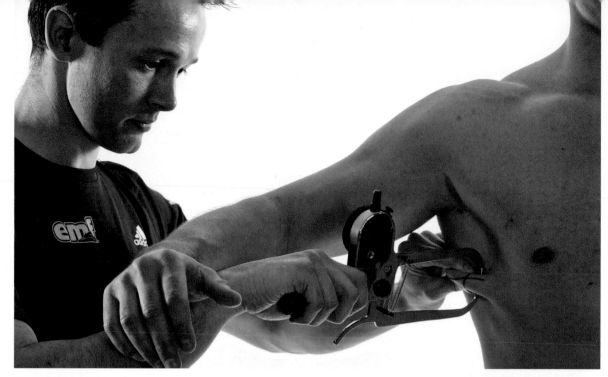

Figure 3.16 Midaxillary measurement

marking another horizontal line and then drawing a diagonal line up through the mark towards the anterior axiallary fold (armpit crease at the front). Take the measure between the two marks on a 45 degree angle down towards the midline of the body.

MIDAXILLARY (BELOW THE ARMPIT)

Locate the xiphoid process (the lower tip of the sternum or breast bone). Make a mark level with this height at the midaxillary point, basically under the armpit halfway between the front and back of the body. Take the pinch vertically at this point.

THIGH

The anterior (front) of the thigh is usually the site used for this although the back can be used in certain instances. Make a mark midway between the hip crease and the patella. Draw through with

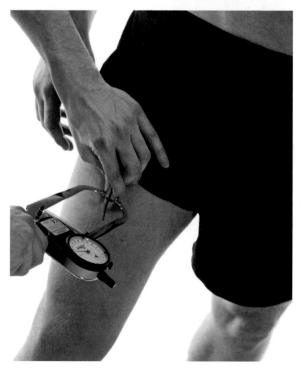

Figure 3.17 Thigh measurement

a vertical line through the belly of the muscle to make a cross and follow the usual measurement procedure.

GASTROCNEMIUS (CALF)

The calf measurement is slightly different in that instead of finding a midpoint between two bony landmarks, you locate the widest point of the calf by measuring the circumference. Once located, take a vertical fold on the medial (inside) of the calf and measure as usual.

Now you know how to take the measurements it's vital you understand what to do with them. Whichever protocol you have used you should add up the recordings you have. Once done you can use a calculation, chart or nomogram to estimate body fat. The latter is a diagram with lines representing different factors such as gender, age and total skinfold measurement that you join up to get your percentage score – a bit like a dot to dot. You can then compare the body fat percentage you have gained to norms charts like the one on page 49 in order to feedback to the client the possible impact on their health and agree goals for improvement if necessary.

Each skinfold protocol has its own formula, but these can involve complex calculations and be very time-consuming. Luckily, these days you can find a host of Internet resources that already have the calculations programmed in for you, allowing you to type in the client's age and gender and the sum of their skinfolds and 'hey presto', you have a percentage body fat reading and haven't had to pretend to be Sir Isaac Newton for the last 20 minutes. An excellent site for this is exrx.net; it allows you to type in scores for three-site and seven-site protocols and estimate body fat percentage.

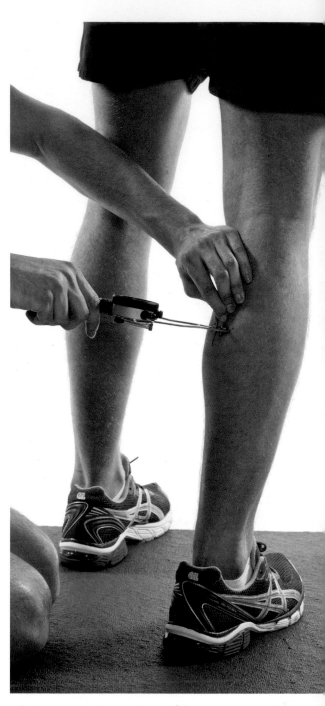

Figure 3.18 Gastrocnemius measurement

Alternatively you can do it without the use of technology using calculations that are readily available. Below is an example of one such equation, created by Jackson and Pollock (1985) for a four-site test using the triceps, abdomen, suprailiac and thigh. There are different equations for men and women.

Men:
Body fat percentage = (0.29288 × total of 4 skinfolds) − (0.0005 × total of 4 skinfolds^2) + (0.15845 × age) + 5.76377

Women:
Body fat percentage = (0.29669 × total of 4 skinfolds) − (0.00043 × total of 4 skinfolds^2) + (0.02963 × age) + 1.4072

For example, William, 28, is a telesales worker who does little exercise and had a four skinfold total of 58. His body fat reading was calculated using the formula above:

(0.29288 × 58 = 16.98704) − (0.0005 × 58^2 = 0.000841) + (0.15845 × 28 = 4.4366) + 5.76377 = 27.18 per cent body fat (excess according to Table 3.7)

Kate, 46, is a marathon runner and had a four skinfold measurement total of 47. Her body fat calculation is shown below:

(0.29669 × 47 = 13.94443) − (0.00043 × 46^2 = 0.00039125) + (0.02963 × 46 = 1.36298) + 1.4072 = 16.71 per cent body fat (very lean according to Table 3.7)

Finally, when you have your body fat percentage you can compare it against the population as a whole. Some people do not like to be classified so this is not essential but others like to know how they measure up and it can help you to set goals to progress from one category to the next. There is no definitive agreed classification as there is with BMI, and what is considered 'normal' or 'ideal' varies with gender and age and from study to study. Table 3.7 can act as a guide, but the focus should be on ensuring good health measures in terms of blood pressure, cholesterol, etc., and in ensuring the client is happy and comfortable with their size and shape.

Table 3.7	Body fat percentage categories	
Category	**Male**	**Female**
Very lean/athletic	6–10%	12–18%
Healthy	11–18%	19–25%
Acceptable	19–24%	26–31%
Excess	25% +	32% +

For clients, a healthy level of body fat is generally the suggested target, and athletes should be educated as to the risks associated with being very lean, particularly irregularities with the menstrual cycle for females.

Now you know how to carry out the two most commonly used measurements, BIA and skinfold testing and you can compare the results to enable you to offer guidance to clients. It's likely you'll be choosing between the two methods, so Table 3.8 gives you a useful summary of the pros, cons and considerations of each.

Table 3.8   Pros and cons of BIA and skinfold testing

Measurement method	Benefits	Drawbacks	Considerations
BIA	• Quick and easy to administer • Not invasive as they can be handheld or at the very most involve the removal of shoes and socks • Basic measuring devices these days are relatively cheap and widely available.	• Lots of variables affect the readings; these include hydration levels, lifestyle in recent days, hand and foot positioning and, if using sensors, the placement of these on the skin • Some models of device deemed higher quality can be expensive • Cannot be used for pregnant women or those fitted with pacemakers	• Clients should ideally fast for four hours prior to the test • No exercise should be carried out for 12 hours prior to the test • No caffeine or alcohol should be consumed before the reading • The menstrual cycle can affect the results so for women time of the month should be factored in
Skinfold measurements	• If administered accurately the readings can be very reliable • Basic calipers are cheap • Three- or four-site measurements can be done fairly quickly	• More accurate calipers can become costly (around £150–200) • Clients must remove clothing to enable the tests to be carried out • Testing more sites takes a long time and leaves greater margin for error • If two different people take the tests over time there is likely to be more room for error in the results	• Ask yourself if you need this level of accuracy with clients? Athletes may do; the general public probably don't • Practice a lot before you do it for real to ensure you are accurate • Think about where you'll carry this out, you'll need somewhere private for people to remove clothing but also consider offering your client the chance to invite a friend/ partner to protect you against allegations of misconduct

Client Case Study:

Sarah was overweight and had taken on a personal trainer, Katie, to help her lose weight. She had some body issues and was low in confidence. Katie and Sarah agreed after having not one but two consultations to make Sarah feel at ease and comfortable, that they would arrange an assessment session. Katie explained to Sarah that she would talk her through each of the different possible measurements and that she could decide whether or not she wished to have them carried out. Katie explained that Sarah could ask questions at any time and that if she did not feel comfortable they could stop a test at any point. She also offered Sarah the opportunity to have her husband or a friend there if that would make her more comfortable.

On the day, Katie went through each of the tests, explaining the purpose, how they would be done, what the results would mean and asking if Sarah had any questions. Sarah was happy to have her circumference measurements taken and was interested in the importance of the location of body fat. She felt it was useful to be able to track changes in her shape and size over time, as her goal was to get into a smaller dress size. Sarah was not comfortable being weighed and did not want to remove clothing to have skinfold tests carried out. She was however happy to use a handheld BIA device to get an estimate of her body fat. Katie explained that these were not necessarily 100 per cent accurate but that they could serve as a useful guide and could be repeated every month or so, to track Sarah's progress.

Sarah was happy at the end of the session that she had some starting points to work from and said that she did not find the assessments anywhere near as daunting as she had imagined.

OTHER WAYS TO MEASURE BODY FAT

Ranging from using height and body circumferences through to complex machinery, scientists are forever finding new ways to estimate body composition. A few of them are reviewed briefly here.

HYDROSTATIC WEIGHING

Sometimes referred to as 'underwater weighing', this describes it nicely. Usually the person tested is placed in a chair and then completely submerged into a special tank. A person will weigh less under water than they do out of it and the difference can be used to calculate how much of an individual's body is fat and how much is other tissues, such as muscle and bone. Complex calculations enable this and take into account factors such as air left in the lungs.

Hydrostatic weighing machines are usually only found in laboratories, are expensive and the protocol is complex and time-consuming so although very accurate, it is unlikely to be used unless for research or for athletes needing accurate clinical measures.

BOD POD

This works in a similar way to hydrostatic weighing, but instead of water, it measures air displacement. The calculation takes into account the volume of air in the pod, a special machine, before the subject enters it, and the volume of air once they are inside. The difference is used to estimate body fat. It is a relatively quick test to carry out at around five to ten minutes, but the equipment is extremely costly.

DEXA SCANS

To give it its full title, dual-energy X-ray absorptiometry uses two X-rays fired at different energy levels through the body. Primarily it is used to measure bone density but it can also be used for body composition. It's known to have a good degree of accuracy and takes just over ten minutes to carry out, but again it's the equipment costs and space required that make it more useful to the medical world than to fitness.

MRI SCANS

Magnetic resonance imaging, or MRI scans use a combination of radio waves and magnetic fields to create pictures of the human body. They are used for numerous reasons in the health world but have become renowned for their accuracy in assessing body composition. They can measure body fat percentage, muscle mass, bone mass and also the location of internal fat, including visceral fat around the organs. This makes it a fantastic tool for detailed medical investigation and for highly accurate readings, but the cost of the machines (at anywhere between £100,000 second-hand up to £2 million) means you're unlikely to see them in a gym anytime soon.

OTHER FITNESS TESTS

Although you may primarily be working with a client to help them change shape or reduce their body fat levels, you may also consider using other assessments to measure the different components of fitness.

WHY DO THIS?

You may want to get an idea of a person's physical ability in order to set an exercise programme at the right level for them or to set appropriate goals. As an instructor, you may also want think about how being overweight has affected your client's cardiovascular fitness, muscular strength and endurance, flexibility, functional ability and balance. This will give you an idea of what to focus on in the exercise sessions.

CARDIOVASCULAR FITNESS

With overweight and obese clients there are many considerations to be made. Firstly, are they otherwise healthy individuals or have they been referred through an exercise referral scheme and have other conditions to be aware of?

If the latter then, dependent on the other conditions, you may not even test, or you would choose a very low level assessment such as a five-minute walk.

Even for those without comorbidities, lower level testing is more appropriate. High impact exercise, such as jogging, places great strain on the joints, in particular the ankles, knees, hips and spine. When running, between three and five times the bodyweight goes through the joints, meaning that for someone weighing 15 stone, (210 pounds), the equivalent of 45–75 stone (630–1,050 pounds) of pressure can be placed through the body. General conditioning is poor in obese individuals and with their increased risk of coronary heart disease it means that submaximal tests are more appropriate. Those who are obese may also overheat more quickly even at low levels of intensity, balance may be altered due to changes in centre of gravity meaning that treadmills should be used cautiously, and general confidence may mean that challenging tests may be intimidating and impact adherence.

You can choose from the following tests:

- Step tests – simple, submaximal step-up protocols such as the YMCA three-minute test, the Chester or Harvard step tests (all of which can be easily found by typing the relevant name into an internet search engine) can be used to estimate VO_2 max (the amount of oxygen taken in over one minute) or recovery rate, both of which can be used as markers of fitness.
- Walk tests – the Rockport walking test, single-stage treadmill test, or six-minute walk test may be appropriate choices. Alternatively, walk tests can be devised to suit an individual. Choose a suitable length of time or a distance to measure any number of variables including 'rate of perceived exertion' (RPE), heart rate, biomechanical or gait analysis and functional ability.
- Seated/recumbent bike tests – the recumbent bike can be an excellent choice because of its comfortable seat and back support. Again, a protocol such as the Astrand test may be applied or a measure of distance, time and exertion can be recorded.

One measure very useful to take with less conditioned clients is the 'preferred rate of perceived exertion'. In essence you use the Modified Borg (CR10) Scale (Borg, 1998) and conduct a graded submaximal test with your client, gradually increasing the intensity up to a level that is safe, likely up to a maximum of five or six, equivalent to hard exercise where the client will be sweaty and a little breathless. Throughout the test, monitor the level (speed and incline if using a treadmill), RPE, heart rate if you wish and any other visual or verbal cues as to the level of effort such as sweat rate, colour, breathing rate and posture.

Cool the client down gradually after completion and then ask them about the level at which they felt most comfortable during the exercise. This is not meant to be clinically validated, rather it can help to give you an idea of where your client feels most comfortable during exercise and ensure you judge the intensity of sessions to challenge them without making them feel uncomfortable. As clients get fitter over time, you may find that they start to feel comfortable working at harder intensities and that the RPE they report at any given heart rate is lower than when they first started.

Many believe that early gym sessions for clients should be about getting them fit, but arguably developing an exercise habit and ensuring people feel safe, comfortable and enjoy their experience is the key. Fitness can build over time, but if they give up then of course it won't.

TESTS OF FUNCTION, ENDURANCE, STRENGTH, FLEXIBILITY AND MOBILITY

Traditional tests of muscle strength and endurance involve repetition maximums, performed on a range of exercises and with rep ranges chosen dependent on the goals or experience of the client. Heavy repetition maximum testing is unlikely to be useful or advised in many cases with overweight or obese clients due to the fact that many will be deconditioned, and high intensity exercise creates unnecessary risks. This type of exercise early in their routines would intimidate many and it would be of little use to the instructor in designing exercise programmes. This is not to say that resistance training is not useful, far from it, as you will see in Chapter 6. The focus should however be on improving mobility and function for everyday movements.

The sit to stand test assesses strength and endurance in the legs and core muscles, and has great carry-over to life as many adults struggle with tasks like getting in and out of a chair as they get older. Studies have shown that obesity can cause changes in posture and movement during sit to stand tasks that may increase the risk of injury in the long term (Sibella et al, 2003). This means you can assess not only strength and endurance, but also posture and functional ability at the same time through close observation of technique.

Step 1:

Place a chair against a wall to ensure that it cannot move or fall backwards during the test. Have the client sit towards the front third of the chair. It should be at such a height that the thighs are parallel to the floor when seated. Feet should be flat on the floor hip to shoulder width apart, arms across the body to prevent using them to assist the lift.

Step 2:

The client should attempt to stand with good posture being maintained throughout.

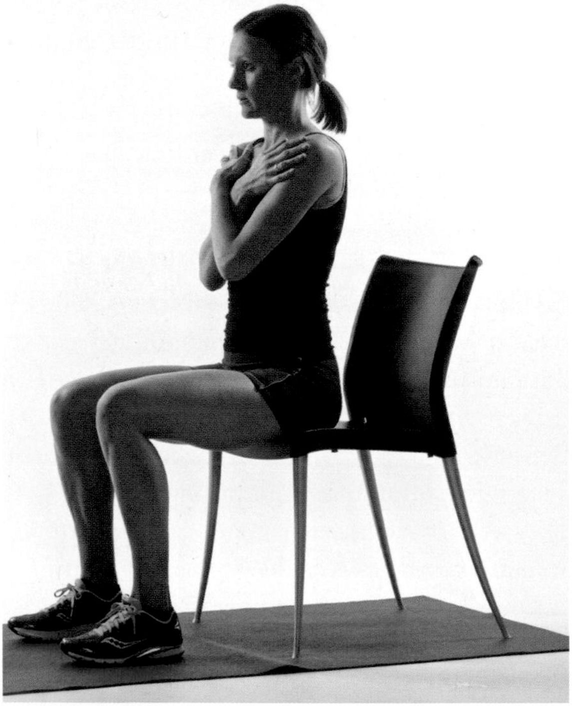

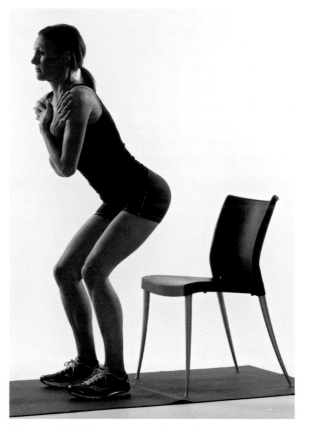

Figure 3.19 Sit to stand test, step 1

Figure 3.20 Sit to stand test, step 2

Step 3:

If the client can do this, they should lower themselves gently and repeat.

Step 4:

Continue the test until the client feels they wish to stop or the technique falters. Record the number of repetitions.

This can be a repetition maximum test, or timed – the latter is often used for older clients, in which case 30 seconds is the timeframe generally accepted. It uses body weight and everyday movements, so is extremely relevant to assess normal functioning. For your more elderly clients you can use the table on the next page to show how their functional ability compares against others in their age range. Anything below these scores is considered below average and suggests a need for improvement.

Remember you can always adapt a test to make it suitable to an individual if needed. For example, for the sit to stand test, use a higher chair, starting with thighs slightly above parallel if required, or

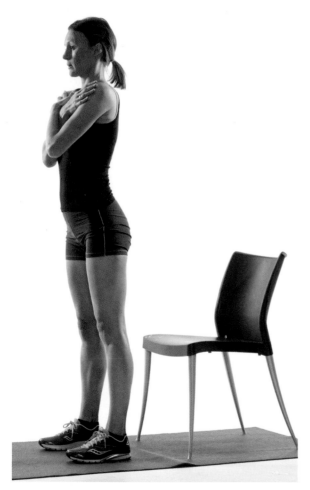

Figure 3.21 Sit to stand test, step 3

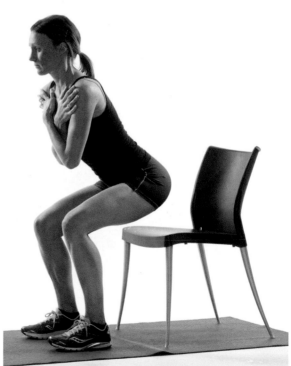

Figure 3.22 Sit to stand test, step 4

Table 3.9	Norms for the 30-second sit to stand test	
Age (years)	Male	Female
60–64	14	12
65–69	12	11
70–74	12	10
75–79	11	10

(adapted from the US Centre for Disease Control and Prevention (2013))

use one with arm supports if necessity demands. As long as you repeat the protocol each time then you can track changes, you just can't use the norms to compare to. Other exercises may be used to test strength and endurance but consider whether the data gained is relevant. Do you need to know how many chest presses they can do? Will it benefit your programming?

Overweight and obese clients may frequently have impaired flexibility and mobility. As such, some form of testing may be considered to measure this and track improvement over time. Again, ask yourself if you need to do it. Will it offer you useful information above what you already know? Are the risks of the tests outweighed by the benefits? Is the client comfortable having the tests carried out?

Choose from the following as appropriate:

VISUAL TESTS

A simple test is to perform basic stretches and record the range of motion the client achieves. This can be recorded using photographs if the client is comfortable with this. Whatever you do don't start snapping away without their knowledge or permission. Stretches for most of the major muscles can be turned into tests. See the examples below for how tape measures can be used to assess range of movement.

Hamstrings

Some overweight clients find it challenging getting up and down from the floor so use a chair-based hamstrings stretch and measure the distance between their fingertips and their toes when they lean forwards. Clients should sit on the front third of the chair. Ensure they maintain a decent posture to prevent strain on their back, flexing from the hips. Clients should place hands on top of one another when leaning forwards and ease gently into the stretch, holding it for around two seconds before the recording is taken. You should instruct them to breathe out gently as they move into the stretch. Repeat for both legs. Scores are recorded based on centimetres, as either a minus score if the hand does not reach the toes or a plus score for any reading past the toes (Jones and Rikli, 2002).

Norms for this test have at present only been designed for elderly clients so the best way to track progress is to record the initial score and measure progress through increases in flexibility.

Chest

Ask your client to place their palms on the base of their back and squeeze their elbows together to the point of mild discomfort. Measure the distance between the tips of the elbows.

Shoulder mobility

Ask your clients to place one arm behind their back and the other over their shoulder as in Figure 3.25.

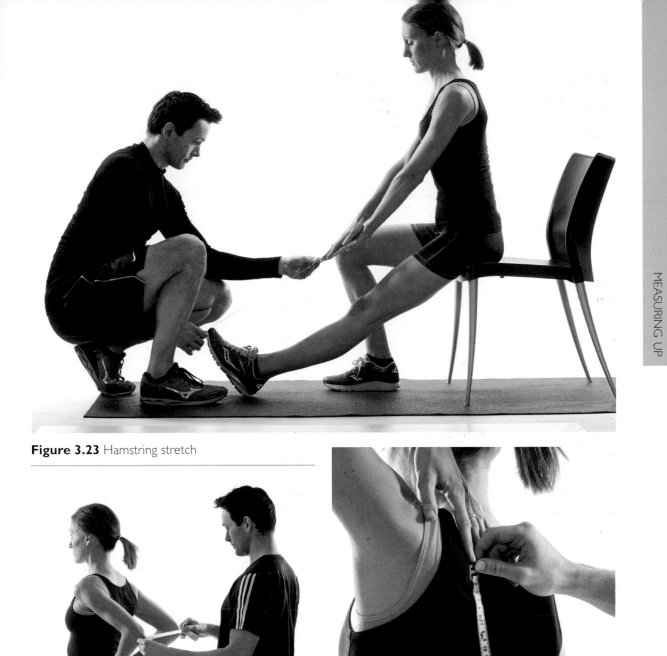

Figure 3.23 Hamstring stretch

Figure 3.24 Chest stretch

Figure 3.25 Shoulder mobility

57

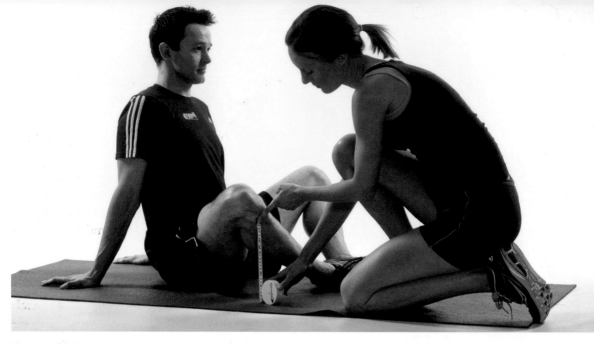

Figure 3.26 Adductors stretch

Measure the distance between the fingertips and then repeat on the other side. It should be possible to get the middle digits of the hands to touch. If the test causes discomfort do not perform it, you already know that you need to work on mobility so simply add stretches to the exercise programme and then repeat the test again further down the line. If there is no discomfort you can begin to take readings and progress from there. If the client feels pain and shows signs or symptoms of injury, refer to a physiotherapist.

Adductors

Sit on the floor, soles of the feet together as close to the body as is comfortable. Note this distance to ensure repeatability when the test is next performed. Drop the legs down to the floor as far as feels comfortable and record the distance between the bony protuberance on the outside of the knee and the floor. Do this for both sides and measure improvements over time.

GONIOMETRY

Essentially a giant protractor, a goniometer is used to measure degrees of movement possible at a joint. This makes it more clinically accurate than the tests described above, but as with skinfold measurements it takes a high degree of accuracy and skill. The equipment is cheap and tests can be quickly administered.

MOTOR SKILLS TESTING

Balance can be affected by changes in posture and centre of gravity that occur with weight gain and as such may need to be tested. Many balance tests are simple to administer, just consider the client's risk for falls and level of confidence before choosing the most appropriate.

Single-leg stand

As the name suggests, ask the client to stand on one leg and record the time in seconds that they can maintain this with good posture and

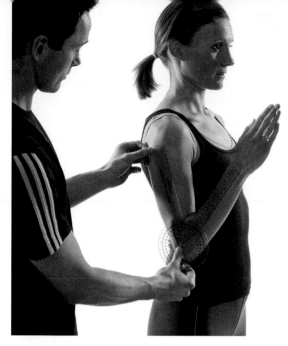

Figure 3.27 Goniometry

without moving the standing leg. Repeat on both sides. Some may find this challenging, so consider having them stand by a wall to hold on to if required or choose a simpler test.

For more elderly clients adapting the single-leg test to have the other foot on tiptoes or even feet together as in a two-leg stand test. This could be performed for up to two minutes.

Heel-to-toe walks

Ask the client to walk along a straight line placing one heel against the toe of the other foot each time.

STRUCTURING AN ASSESSMENT SESSION

You now have a range of tests to choose from in your toolkit. The skill comes in working out which ones to use with your clients. Each person will have a different set of needs and you should think about the following when deciding the structure of your testing sessions:

- Client comfort – what are they happy to have done? Are they happy to have physical contact? Do they wish to have a friend/partner present for the testing?
- Environment – how much space do you have to carry out the tests? How much privacy is available?
- Equipment – how much kit do you have? How costly is it to buy new materials? How long does the equipment take to use? How much training do you require to use them accurately?
- Repeatability – can you carry out the same tests over time to ensure you get an accurate marker of progress?
- Validity – are the tests you have chosen useful for the outcomes you are trying to achieve?

Once you've agreed on the tests with your client, set up the session professionally by providing them with advice about what they should and shouldn't do beforehand, for example abstaining from caffeine and exercise. Offer them an outline of what will happen before they arrive to set their expectations.

Upon arrival, spend some time chatting with the client to increase rapport and put them at ease. This is known as small talk for a reason, so keep it light, and you should spend a good few minutes doing this before progressing to the 'big talk' of the actual tests. When you do, ask if they have any questions or concerns before you get into the actual testing. If they do, take time to respond to these and adjust the structure of the session if needed. This session structure was suggested to me by a man called Keith Smith, an expert in the fitness industry in working with deconditioned clients or those new to exercise. Keith has been heavily involved over the years in focusing on the importance of soft skills when working with clients in a fitness setting and has a wealth of experience in delivering to clients who may require additional support to successfully achieve their goals.

Once you are ready to begin the tests, it is important to consider the order. You should have already completed a medical questionnaire but if not do so before doing anything else. Tests can be performed in a variety of orders but an outline is suggested below:

- Blood glucose/cholesterol – if you happen to be doing this, get it out of the way. People are often most nervous about this and they will have fasted for eight hours so will be hungry. Once the tests are done they will be able to have a snack before continuing so remind them to bring something to eat.
- Blood pressure – again this can make people nervous and if you are not doing finger-prick tests, this should likely be your starting point. Should the client have a high reading initially, especially the systolic (higher) pressure then you have time to let them relax before repeating it later.
- Height and weight – these are commonly known tests and simple and quick to carry out. You can calculate BMI at this point and then explain its upsides and limitations, which can lead you nicely into other measurements. If using BIA scales you will be able to take the body fat reading at this point too.
- Circumferences – take waist, hips and other body measurements as agreed with your client.
- Skinfolds – you can emphasise the importance

of body fat and then draw together all of the results to offer the client a detailed picture of their current status.
- Active tests – if performing other fitness tests the order depends on those chosen but in general you may perform a submaximal cardiovascular test to warm up your client and then follow it with functional, mobility, motor skill and flexibility tests.

At every stage, ask if they are happy, provide the opportunity for them to ask anything they wish to, and explain things simply in a language they understand. Ensure they are fully aware of why each test is important to them and what the results they achieve mean. After the session, make sure you provide your client with a copy of the results in a simple format that they can use to chart their progress over time.

SUMMARY
- Health screening is essential prior to delivering sessions for overweight and obese clients to ensure they are safe to exercise.
- A range of tests are available to track changes in shape and weight. Appropriate tests should be chosen for the individual and the benefits and drawbacks explained.
- Other tests of fitness and function may also be useful to set goals, develop programmes and monitor progress.
- Soft skills are an essential part of the testing process as assessments can be intimidating.

GOAL SETTING AND BEHAVIOUR CHANGE

4

Goal setting is important for all clients so it's necessary for you to know how to agree goals and what excellent targets look like. Overweight clients may have many things stopping them achieving their targets and so it's vital to have plans in place to overcome these, especially as you know how few people seem to succeed in their weight loss attempts. The key comes in setting up an environment that allows people to change behaviour permanently. Next we look at the various change models available to help you.

WEIGHING UP YOUR OPTIONS

Clients may often say 'I want to lose some weight'. OK, that's a good start, but how much, why, by when, how will they know when they've lost what they want? Without clear goal setting, it's hard to quantify and measure achievements, or to know when the target is reached. At what point will they be satisfied? Is there anything else they want?

As an instructor you need to be able to motivate people, and proving that change has taken place is an effective way of doing this. Equally, discovering that no progress has been made is just as useful and can act as a kick-start for some, or

at least offer the opportunity to discuss a change of approach. You must also remember that, be it a gym or personal training session, people are paying for this service and expect to get results. This is not to say that it's down to you to achieve for them, on the contrary, you need to emphasise to clients that you will support and advise them but that ultimately it's what they do that makes the difference. You need to be determined in your efforts to help bring about the changes they desire, and to be absolutely clear about exactly what those changes are. By working with clients to discover their precise expectations, you'll be able to find out quickly whether or not these are realistic and to use your knowledge and skills to explain to them what sensible aims are and to adjust and agree targets as necessary.

There are a range of approaches that can be taken to set goals but there are common strands that run throughout. These include clarity of the goal, setting timeframes, assessing the reality of the goal and agreeing how you're going to measure its success. Two researchers called Locke and Latham (2006) have spent years researching goals and have identified that if they are to be truly motivational for people they must have a number of features. These include:

Difficulty: research shows that goals must be hard enough to motivate people. If they are too easy, motivation levels decrease as people achieve a greater sense of satisfaction from a challenging goal.

Specificity: they note that vague goals, such as 'I want to lose some weight', 'I want to tone up a bit' or 'I want to get a bit fitter' achieve lower levels of success than those that are detailed and precise, for example 'I want to lose five pounds' or 'I want to get into a size 10 dress'. They also suggest that the effectiveness of goal setting is influenced by a number of things. These are:

- Feedback – people need to be able to both give and receive feedback about how they are doing, and use this to judge whether amendments to goals are required.
- Commitment – people must buy in to the goal they are working towards. People can set goals themselves, agree them with someone, or have outcomes set for them, but they must actually want to do it for them to be effective.
- Complexity – it must be hard enough to be challenging but not so hard that it either cannot be achieved, or can but only at the expense of other things important to them.

This research links very nicely into two of the well-known goal setting models:

- SMART goal setting
- The GROW model

GETTING SMART ABOUT WEIGHT LOSS

Used in everything from top-level sports to big business, from personal training sessions to accountancy, SMART goals are an extremely effective way to structure targets and desires. Let's have a look at what the acronym SMART stands for:

Specific – this tells you exactly what it is your client wants. How much weight do they want to lose? What size clothes do they want to be able to wear? What body fat percentage are they aiming for?

Measurable – now you know what they want, how are they going to know when it has been achieved? Can you track the changes? Progress can be measured using any of the tests in the previous chapter, or even through clothing size.

Agreed or Achievable – there are different versions of the SMART model in circulation. Some talk about the importance of agreeing goals, ensuring that the goal setter has ownership of them and other versions stress the importance of making the goals achievable. Both options have links back to the research by Locke and Latham and as such either can be used and the goal will still be effective.

Realistic or Relevant – again there are some different options available. Realistic shares much in common with achievable goals and so it's best not to use both together to analyse a goal. The other R stands for relevance and is important to consider. What will achieving the goal do? Does it relate closely to other goals and importantly, does it conflict with other goals? If the latter is true, it's best to revisit this as conflicting goals mean that one or the other, or worse still both are unlikely to be achieved. For example, a common goal for men is to lose a fairly substantial amount of weight while also bulking up at the same time. It is not that this is impossible but it is challenging to do both at the same time. It is best to ask your client which goal is the priority, focus on that one first and then move on to the other once it has been achieved.

Time-framed – to know if a goal is achievable/realistic then you need to consider the time-frame. If, as Peter Kay once said in his now infamous stand-up gig, the aim is to lose '14 stone, in a day', then it's unlikely to happen.

Some models use SMARTER which adds the requirement that goals are Enjoyable and Recorded.

People may have a variety of goals. Some may want to change things that are visual, or seemingly simple to measure, such as losing weight or dropping a dress size. While others may have goals that seem less tangible, like having more energy or feeling more confident. None of these goals are any better or more important than the other; it all depends on the individual's values.

Think SMART not HARD

While the science on safe and effective rates of weight loss is sketchy to say the least, there are some general guidelines that may be of use when agreeing realistic timeframes.

If the goal is to lose weight the general recommendation of most medical institutions is to aim for around 1–2 pounds (0.5–1 kg) a week. Some recommend up to 3 pounds per week and this may certainly be the case for those new to exercise or with more to lose. For obese clients, rates of weekly weight loss above this may dramatically increase the risk of gallstones (Weinsier et al, 1995). Other than this, the science on these recommendations is somewhat limited, and is based more on the fact that research shows that rapid weight loss is often not sustained in the long term.

In terms of body fat, there are no clear guidelines on how much can be lost in a given time, possibly because it really depends on the fat percentage and fitness of the individual at the outset. From experience, an average of 1–3 per cent body fat can be lost in the early months of exercise, slowing as a person gets closer to healthier ranges.

Changes in circumference measurements are specific to individuals and how much can be lost in a given time is hard to predict. Sensible goals such as 1–2 centimetres off areas such as the waist are attainable in the early stages but you can adapt goals regularly with clients based on their progress. Over the years the notion that it is possible to lose weight from one specific area, known as 'spot-reducing' has been refuted as myth. It's a concept that's been peddled from as far back as the 1960s with one study showing that fat loss was noted in one arm when performing resistance training on it for six weeks while the other arm remained the same having done no training (Olson and Edlestein, 1968). In recent years, Charles Poliquin (2013) has suggested, based on data he has collected in his work, that fat storage in certain areas may be due to hormonal imbalances and that, by correcting these, spot reduction is possible. This has gained popularity in the industry and it is certainly worthy of further research.

You could classify goals as being:

- Physical appearance related – changes in shape or size.
- Health related – to decrease future risk of disease or to manage a current medical condition.
- Social – goals may be about having fun or spending time with family and friends, or to make new ones.
- Psychological – someone may want to feel happier or have more energy.
- Fitness/physiological – to increase speed, distance, sports performance, strength or flexibility.
- Functional – similar to fitness, but some may want to improve their ability to do everyday tasks such as climbing the stairs, gardening or getting to and from the shops.

Do not assume that somebody who is overweight will always have a physical appearance goal. They may well have, but often there may be a more important motivator that underpins this and that is often the true goal. If you can build good rapport with people they may feel comfortable to share this with you. For example, someone may wish to lose weight to be able to play football with their children without feeling tired. In this instance then the real goal is one about energy and family values; the weight loss is just the key that opens up the door.

Some people's goals are positively framed and some negatively. More commonly these may be termed 'carrot' or 'stick' goals, or 'towards' or 'away from' goals. Table 4.1 shows you examples of each and how the same goal can be flipped to be something to work towards or something to steer away from.

There is no right or wrong here, some people are more motivated by driving towards something and some need the fear factor to achieve what they want, or don't want in this case. There is research to suggest that positively framed goals may be more motivational, as threats may not act as motivators for many (Drach-Zahavy and Erez, 2002). Similarly, the feedback given to someone about how they are progressing towards their goals can be positive or negative. Seemingly, some are motivated by knowing that they are doing well, while others increase efforts when negative feedback is given that reflects the fact that they are failing to achieve what they want (Fishbach et al, 2010).

What does this all mean for you? If your client has a negatively framed goal, you may want to

Table 4.1	Carrot and stick goals
Carrot or 'towards' goals	**Stick or 'away from' goals**
I want to feel happier and healthier	I don't want to get ill in the future
I want to be able to run for half an hour without stopping	I don't want to feel so unfit
I want to be thinner and fit into my old clothes again	I don't want to be fat any more

work to 'flip it' to a positive one. However, before you do you'll want to ask what motivates them and what sort of feedback they want from you in case they are someone who is effectively motivated by negative goals.

YOUR TURN

If you've not worked with SMART goals before, or you're using this book to help you make your own changes, use the list below to set a target and ensure it meets all of the SMART criteria.

Write down a goal, or goals that you have.

Now check that it is SMART by answering the following questions:

1. Is it specific? Do you know exactly what you want?
2. Can you measure it? How will you do this?
3. Is it achievable? What is it that makes you sure you can do it?
4. What makes it relevant? Why is it important to you? What will it give you?
5. Have you got a timeframe for achieving your goal? Does this fit in with ensuring it is realistic?

STOP SIGNS, ROADBLOCKS AND HURDLES

Everyone who has a goal has barriers or obstacles that make it harder to achieve. It's best to attempt to identify these at the outset in order to make contingency plans. That way, when the issue arises, the person will feel empowered to be able to do something about it. There will be hundreds of ways that potential barriers can be overcome, so it is important to let your client

come up with the best solutions for them. You can act as a sounding board and offer advice if required. Once agreed, these should be recorded so that if and when the barrier appears, the plan can be referred to.

Common barriers for those trying to lose weight include:

- Self-confidence/self-esteem — some may feel uncomfortable exercising in a gym environment due to their appearance or lack of fitness. It is not uncommon to hear people say 'I'm too unfit to join the gym'.
- Medical conditions — as you've seen, being overweight is linked to an increased risk of many illnesses and these may make it more challenging for people to achieve their goals.
- Mood – many will find that there is something that causes them to choose poor foods. This may be mood, for example anger, tiredness, stress or nerves.
- Environment – some will say they can eat well at home but struggle at work or vice versa, or it may be that weekends are their barrier or possibly time spent with family or friends. Each person's environmental barriers will be unique to them.
- Lack of energy — carrying around excess weight is a strain on the body and this should be recognised. While it is known that exercise can improve energy levels, in the early stages it can be hard for extremely overweight people to do enough to make a difference to weight.
- Motivation — some may say that they are not motivated enough to work towards their goal. While you can help by working with them to find out what motivates them, ultimately it is up to the individual to decide if

Table 4.2	Decisional balance table	
	Benefits	**Drawbacks**
Changing/achieving goals	e.g. more energy to play sports with the children	e.g. won't be able to eat the foods I enjoy regularly
Staying the same	e.g. don't have to make any major life changes	e.g. will still be overweight and feel tired a lot of the time

they wish to make changes. You can use the decisional balance table above to see if the person is ready to work towards their goals. If the benefits of change and the drawbacks of staying the same outweigh the answers in the opposing boxes by number or importance to the client then they are ready for change. If not you can discuss with them what would need to happen for them to be ready and support these changes if possible. If they perceive staying as they are as the better option then that is their choice and should be respected. That said, you should educate clients about the benefits of change if they are unaware of them.

THE GROW MODEL

Linked closely to SMART goal setting is the GROW model, a coaching tool that allows you to look at how changes can be implemented and it can be very useful when working with weight loss or health goals. GROW stands for:

Goals – what do you want? SMART can certainly be used here to link the two models together.

Reality – where are you now? This links back to the consultation and health-screening already discussed.

Obstacles/Options – the obstacles are the barriers in the way and the options the ways in which these can be overcome.

Will – this is the stage where you establish the desire from the person to make the changes. You may use the decisional balance table to ensure the person is ready to change, or you may ask questions such as 'So you know what you want to do now, can you make those changes?' and 'If yes, will you make the changes? What will you do first?' You may also use scales to check someone's desire to change, such as 'On a scale of 0–10, with 10 being most important, how important is it for you to make the changes we have discussed?' 'How likely are you on a scale of 0–10 to make those changes?' These are common questioning techniques used in behaviour change methodologies like NLP (neurolinguistic programming) and motivational interviewing.

Various coaching methodologies and systems have been developed over the past century and the interest in this aspect of psychology has boomed in the past 30 years or so. Some of these have been used for health and fitness goals in recent times.

NLP (Neurolinguistic Programming)

NLP uses a variety of tools and techniques to look at the links between how people think, the language they use and how they act. Richard Bandler and John Grinder originally developed it from their own work in the field and through their experience of the works of other psychologists, including Milton Erickson.

MI (Motivational Interviewing)

Developed initially by Stephen Rollnick and William Miller, MI is a counselling technique using open questions, reflective listening and other methods to allow people to work out how to motivate themselves to make changes and achieve goals.

I GET BY WITH A LITTLE HELP FROM MY FRIENDS

Identifying a support network is a crucial part of achieving goals. As the Beatles once said, 'I get by with a little help from my friends' and Bill Withers shared the view by telling us that 'we all need somebody to lean on'.

SO WHAT IS THE ROLE OF A SUPPORT NETWORK?

Some people may need a motivator, others may need someone to physically do something for them such as join in with exercise sessions, drive them to and from the gym, look after the children so that they can have time to exercise, help with the cooking or buy the right foods at the supermarket. It's all about helping the person to make the changes they've identified, whether it is emotional or physical support.

WHO SHOULD BE IN THE SUPPORT NETWORK?

Common members of support networks include:

- Family – husbands, wives, brothers and sisters, parents, children and extended family may all play a part.
- Friends – old pals, neighbours, those in the social circle, gym buddies and anyone else from important groups who can help in some way.
- Professionals – fitness instructors and personal trainers, medical practitioners like GPs, nurses, physiotherapists, dieticians or counsellors may all have a part to play depending on the situation.

DO SUPPORT NETWORKS HELP?

James House (1987) suggests that 'social networks', a term we are all more familiar with these days since the coming of Facebook and other sites, play an important role in the health and well-being of individuals. Of course he wasn't specifically referring to Twitter, or any other Internet site, but to the importance of any group of people close to an individual. His notion has been backed up more recently by research that suggests that people's health is better and risks for mortality are decreased when they have social networks that offer emotional support (Uchino, 2006).

HOW DO YOU BUILD A SUPPORT NETWORK?

It doesn't have to be complicated. Ask your client to write down a list of the people they think they will need help from in order to achieve their goals. They should also identify how the person will help them and specify exactly what it is they would like them to do. They should then discuss this with the person to ensure they are happy to help.

MODELS OF BEHAVIOUR CHANGE

Goal setting and overcoming barriers is ultimately about changing behaviour in the long term. This is a difficult thing to achieve, and certainly in the context of weight loss the science shows that while many can lose weight, it is much harder to keep it off. One analysis of various studies suggests that only 20 per cent of people who managed to lose at least 10 per cent of their starting weight kept it off after a year (Wing and Phelan, 2005).

As fitness professionals, your priority should be to work with individuals to make sustainable life changes. There are a few models of change that you may find useful to help with this, but before we look at them, let's take the time to define what behaviour change means.

The National Institute for Health and Clinical Excellence (NICE, 2007) define behaviour as 'the product of individual or collective human actions, seen within and influenced by their structural, social and economic context'. So behaviour change refers to a sustained or permanent alteration in these actions.

STAGES OF CHANGE MODEL

Also known as the trans-theoretical model, this was developed by Prochaska and DiClemente in the 1970s and has since been adapted to become the model used today. Originally used to relate to smoking and alcohol cessation, it was taken on by the fitness industry because of its relationship to health and its relatively easy to follow nature.

The model consists of various stages of change that a person can progress or regress through. Each stage represents how ready to make changes an individual is at any given time. The stages, in order are:

Pre-contemplation

At this stage, an individual is not considering making lifestyle changes any time soon. They may be aware that their current lifestyle is unhealthy but not want to change, or they may not even understand that what they are doing may have negative consequences in the future.

Contemplation

A person in this stage is considering making changes to their lifestyle at some point in the next six months. They have thought about the benefits of changing but still may not be fully convinced that it is the right thing to do.

Preparation

Having thought it through, the individual is ready to make changes and begins to get ready to do so. They intend to begin the changes in the next month.

Action

The person is making changes to their lifestyle, having started within the last six months. They are consistently managing to behave in the new way and are motivated to achieve what they want. If a person is not acting out these changes consistently, they should be classified as being in the preparation stage.

Maintenance

The person has managed to commit to the change and keep it up regularly for a period of six months or more.

Termination

This sounds negative but in fact it's the exact opposite. Termination refers to the point at which the change becomes a permanent part of the person's lifestyle, with very little intention of reverting back to old behaviours. With the original purpose of the model being about smoking and alcohol cessation, this stage had real relevance, but with changes to activity levels and eating patterns, this may be less so. Even the most ardent fitness enthusiast may have the odd bad meal or miss a few sessions because of events in life, but this is not really equivalent to having a cigarette, or reverting back to drink.

Relapse

At any stage of the model (except for pre-contemplation), the person can slip backwards. This is known as a relapse. In the fitness world it is common for somebody to join a gym, do a few sessions and then give up, or they'll buy an exercise bike for the home which very soon becomes a convenient place to hang their washing.

If using this model, you need to know how you can help your clients to progress from one stage to the next. The table on the next page gives you a range of ideas that may be helpful.

STRENGTHS AND WEAKNESSES OF THE MODEL

The Stages of Change model offers a nice way of showing progress towards making behavioural changes. The stage-by-stage approach allows people to see how they are doing over time in a fairly simple manner.

There are some weaknesses too though; it could be argued that a person could be in various stages at the same time for exercise, diet and other lifestyle considerations. For example, someone could exercise regularly but be a smoker with no intention of giving up at the present time. This is not a bad thing, it just means that you may have to work through each one individually, identifying what stage they're at and agreeing a way to progress if needed. Some have suggested that people don't always move through the stages in a linear fashion, often jumping straight from contemplation into action or relapsing from action maybe as far back as pre-contemplation.

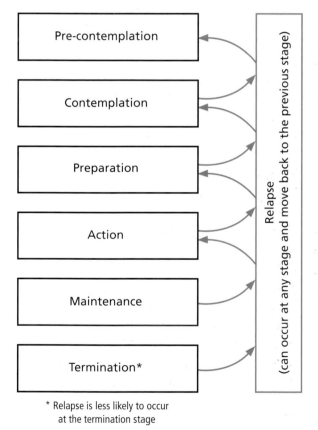

* Relapse is less likely to occur at the termination stage

Figure 4.1 The trans-theoretical model of behaviour change by Prochaska and DiClemente

Table 4.3	Stages of Change model tips
Stage of change	**What can you do?**
Pre-contemplation	• Simply raising the suggestion that change may be required forces somebody to think about it • Educate about the reasons change might be required and also the benefits of making the alterations • Discuss the possible consequences for themselves and for those close to them should they not change
Contemplation	• Complete a decisional balance table like the one on page **66** to assess readiness and desire to make changes • Work with the person to increase the pros of change and decrease the cons. Discuss what they'll get out of changing • Get them to talk to others who've made the changes to gather other opinions • Ask them to talk to family and friends to raise the possibility of change and gather their views and willingness to support if required
Preparation	• This stage may involve health screening and fitness testing to assess the starting point • Agree SMART goals and strategies for overcoming barriers for the changes to come • Ask the person to talk with their support crew about exactly what help they will require • Plan how the changes will be implemented – choose just one or two things to do so as not to overwhelm
Action	• Introduce the interventions; these may be exercise programmes or routines, dietary or other lifestyle changes • Offer support and motivation – this can come in any form the person finds most helpful • Reinforce regularly the benefits of the changes and schedule reviews to check progress and discuss any new barriers
Maintenance	• Continue to support in all of the ways described in the action phase • Set new goals to ensure that there are new challenges to keep the person motivated • Ask them to compare how they think, feel, or look now with when they started • Revisit barriers, pros and cons to ensure no unexpected events can throw the person off track

Table 4.3	Stages of Change model tips (cont.)
Stage of change	**What can you do?**
Relapse	• Should a relapse occur, and it often will, take the time to discuss what action can be taken to get back on track • Go back and review the pros and cons of change; have these changed? Are there now more cons than pros? What can be done to change this? • Revisit goals and barriers • Outline the consequences of not getting back on track, the benefits of picking up again or both (dependent on whether they're a carrot or stick person)

This could certainly be the case with those trying to lose weight but the model can still be of use in guiding and supporting them towards permanent changes.

The science reflects the mixed views on the model, with some success and some failures when used in the context of weight loss. Tuah et al (2011) conducted a review of various studies that had used the model to coach overweight and obese people to lose weight, and found little evidence that it was effective.

However, Johnson et al (2008) carried out a large study on around 1,200 overweight to moderately obese adults. Participants were randomly assigned to either a treatment group who received behaviour change support on exercise, healthy eating and managing emotional eating, or a control group who were left to their own devices. Those who were in pre-contemplation at the start of the study and received the behaviour change support improved in all three areas when compared to those who had no support. Generally, 45–50 per cent of those receiving help had made significant changes and maintained them after two years. This was compared to 30–40 per cent of those who did not have any coaching. Although better than the control group, you could argue that less than half of people making permanent lifestyle changes is not a great number, but compare that to the statistics you've seen already on how few people succeed with weight loss and it stands up quite well. Around a third of the participants who had behaviour change support using the model lost 5 per cent or more of their initial weight and kept it off, compared to 18 per cent who didn't have any support. It clearly doesn't work for everyone, but it may well be worth using as a tool with your clients to increase the chances of success.

OTHER MODELS OF CHANGE

The Stages of Change model is probably most commonly used, but it is not the only one available. You may prefer to use one of the following instead:

THE HEALTH ACTION PROCESS APPROACH

Developed by Ralf Schwarzer, a professor at the Freie University in Berlin, the model has two basic stages:

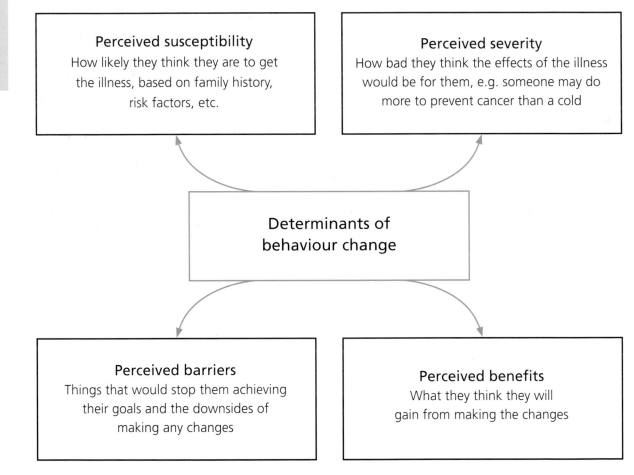

- The motivational (intention to change stage)
- The volitional (planning and doing stage)

Much like Prochaska and DiClemente's model, Schwarzer breaks down changes in behaviour into elements that involve the beginning of an idea that change might be required, through to some form of action to bring it about. What differs is that he takes into account factors that affect whether or not the person will set the goals, such as self-efficacy, the outcomes they expect from making the changes, and the risks they perceive in doing so. The motivational phase is where the goal setting takes place, and the volitional phase is subdivided into pre-action and action phases.

THE HEALTH BELIEF MODEL

This is a very simple model and certainly of some use when working with those who are overweight

Perceived susceptibility
How likely they think they are to get the illness, based on family history, risk factors, etc.

Perceived severity
How bad they think the effects of the illness would be for them, e.g. someone may do more to prevent cancer than a cold

Determinants of behaviour change

Perceived barriers
Things that would stop them achieving their goals and the downsides of making any changes

Perceived benefits
What they think they will gain from making the changes

Figure 4.2 Determinants of behaviour change

or wish to avoid becoming overweight. The model is designed to look at whether or not a person will make a behaviour change that decreases the likelihood of them getting a medical condition, for example diabetes.

It looks at four factors that determine whether or not that person will make a change that would decrease their risk of developing the disease (see Figure 4.2).

THE I-CHANGE MODEL

This model is somewhat of a collage of ideas, taken from the Stages of Change Model, Health Belief Model, goal setting theories and established psychological work by Bandura and Ajzen. It has three basic phases:

- Awareness – the person knows they need to make a change and have a realistic perception of where they are at the present time.
- Motivation – the person becomes intent on making the change.
- Action – the person begins to make the changes. Factors that influence whether or not this occurs are self-efficacy, goal setting, planning and the acquisition of any new skills required to make these changes, for example someone may need to learn to cook in a certain way to eat more healthily.

Regardless of the model used, all are based on the notion of thoughts turning into actions. The key then is to find a way to repeat these actions again and again over time to achieve the outcomes people are looking for.

SUMMARY
- Take the time to set clear goals with people.
- Identify barriers and work to develop ways to overcome them before they become an issue.
- Identify readiness to change and use appropriate strategies with clients to help them make their new behaviour a permanent part of their life.

You've come to the end of the planning phase in this book, and you're ready to begin the action phase, looking at the things people can do to help them lose weight, decrease body fat and improve health.

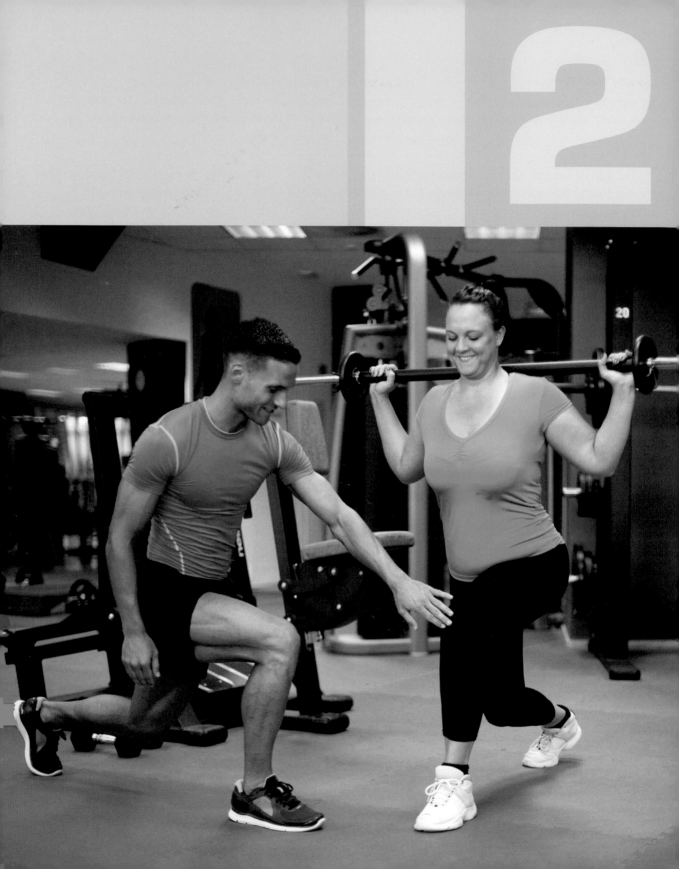

PART **TWO**

MANAGING WEIGHT GAIN AND OBESITY

Successful weight loss and weight management must take a holistic approach; this is evident from the large number of risk factors for weight gain identified earlier. The remaining chapters are dedicated to the things that people can change to achieve a healthy weight. These are diet, exercise and activity, lifestyle and medical interventions including medications and surgery where necessary.

Each of these chapters guides you through current practice and is based on a combination of recommended guidelines and scientific research. Where disagreements exist, the debate is presented to allow you to make your own mind up. As well as providing you with evidence-based research, there are a host of tools supplied for you to use when working with clients. Chapters 5, 6 and 7 include suggested dietary changes, exercises, techniques and programming ideas as well as strategies for improving sleep and managing stress.

Chapter 8 reviews the current medical interventions available and information related to the effectiveness, benefits and risks of these treatments. There follows a wide range of references and resources that you can access to further your knowledge in this area.

// FOOD FOR THOUGHT

THE IMPORTANCE OF DIET

If you had to read just one chapter in this book, this should probably be it. A broad topic to say the least, this chapter looks at two major aspects of diet: *quantity* and *quality* and their relationship to weight loss. Reviewing the science on food intake, I emphasise the importance of portion control and give some useful strategies for achieving this. I also review the information available on the major components of any diet; the macronutrients carbohydrate, fat and protein as well as the different vitamins, minerals and antioxidants, known collectively as micronutrients. The link between food and mood is outlined, and finally I review some of the current popular diets.

Some have claimed that nutrition is the most important factor in effective weight loss and maintenance. A review of weight loss studies using either diet alone, diet and exercise, or exercise alone, found that both methods that included dietary changes were consistently more effective for weight loss, fat loss, decreases in body fat percentage and BMI (Miller et al, 1997). On average, people lost 20–60 per cent less weight using exercise alone.

Interestingly, it may not be about whether diet or exercise plays a more important role, but rather what people believe to be true. Brent McFerran (2013) conducted a large study of nearly 1,200 people across five countries, looking at whether they thought diet or exercise was more important for weight loss. Those who thought diet played a more important role in weight loss consistently had lower BMI scores than those who thought exercise was key. Now there are some weaknesses with this research, it looked at BMI and not body fat, which is a major downfall, but it raises an interesting point. Researchers have suggested that exercising can lead to people overconsuming calories, in fact one study shows that just thinking about exercise caused people to increase food intake (Werle, Wansink and Payne, 2011). McFerran thinks that those who believe diet is more important pay close attention to what they eat but may not exercise as much, whereas those who believe exercise is the key will be more active but may be less strict with their eating. He argues that the exercise group may underestimate how many calories they consume and be unaware of how much activity is required to burn these off.

Regardless of whether exercise or diet is more important, and it's likely that both together offers the best solution, nutrition clearly has a major role to play in weight loss and maintenance.

PLEASE SIR, CAN I HAVE SOME MORE?

It's simple right? You eat too much and don't move around enough and you gain weight, you eat less, move more and you lose weight? This is known as the energy balance equation and is summarised as:

- Calories consumed = calories used = no change in weight
- Calories consumed greater than calories used = weight gain
- Calories used greater than calories consumed = weight loss

There are certain undeniable truths to this equation and calorie intake should be a major consideration for weight loss. It is well-known from studies that overweight people tend to under report the amount of calories they consume (Licthman et al, 1992), and that could clearly play a part in why they are overweight or not losing what they hoped. The difficulty comes in getting the mathematics right, it really isn't that simple to count how many calories are consumed or burned. As you saw in Chapter 2, estimating calorie requirements is just that, an estimate. You're going to need a big abacus if you want clients to record every calorie eaten and used each day. It's just not possible to be this precise unless you have the calorimetry devices available in university science labs. Bear in mind that for thousands of years, mankind did a fairly good job of maintaining a healthy body weight before food labels were invented. Also consider the fact that, in the wild certainly, you don't often see an obese animal. This excludes the rather large pets that have started appearing in the past 30 years

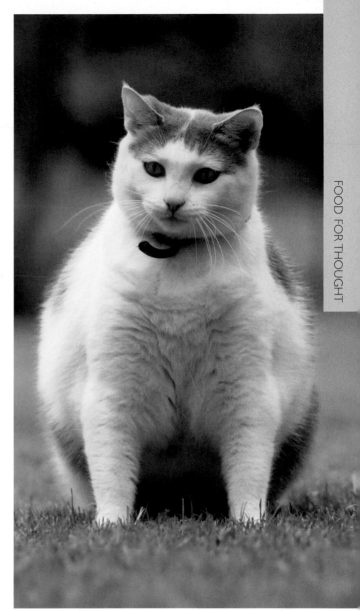

Figure 5.1 Fat cats: even obese pets are now commonplace

or so, probably from sharing their owners' diets of processed convenience foods.

What are calories?

Calories are a measure of the amount of energy in the foods that we eat. To be scientific, they are:

The amount of energy needed to raise the temperature of 1 gram of water by 1 degree Celsius.

Food labels will report the amount of calories contained within, but may use the term kcals or kilocalories; today these are commonly used as an alternative to the term calories.

Calories come from the foods we consume, and different types of food contain different amounts. The macronutrients, or main parts of the diet, carbohydrate, fat and protein, contain approximately:

Carbohydrate: 4 kcals per gram
Fat: 9 kcals per gram
Protein: 4 kcals per gram

So if you want to see how many calories comes from each of these by looking at a food label, you can multiply the number of grams of each by the figures above for a rough guess. These figures are in fact an oversimplification, as different types of fat contain differing amounts of energy but, like all things, they serve as a guide.

THE CURRENT GUIDELINES FOR DAILY CALORIE INTAKE IN THE UK

Table 5.1	Guidelines for daily calorie intake	
Age (years)	Recommended calorie intake (kcals per day)	
	Male	Female
1	765	717
5	1,482	1,362
15	2,820	2,390
18	3,155	2,462
19–24	2,772	2,175
25–34	2,749	2,175
35–44	2,629	2,103
45–54	2,581	2,103
55–64	2,581	2,079
65–74	2,342	1,912
75+	2,294	1,840

Adapted from the Scientific Advisory Committee on Nutrition (2011)

These are useful guidelines for clients but will differ for individuals, based on activity levels, lean mass and other factors.

Rob Dunn of *Scientific American* (Dunn, 2013) suggests that not only is it hard to count calories accurately, but:

- The calories reported on food labels may sometimes be lower than the actual amount consumed, especially in processed foods, with protein and fibre calorie content often being underestimated.

- In 'real' foods the calories reported were at times greater than what was actually taken in, almonds being an example.
- Cooking foods may alter the amount of calories in them that the body absorbs. Also, individual differences in gut bacteria may impact how many calories the body takes in from a given food.

As this is only one study, this research should be taken with a pinch of salt (which luckily has no calories) but it serves to show the complexity of the issues we're dealing with and that just counting calories may not be a good choice. Something that illustrates this well is a news piece from the Mail Online (2009); it was reported that a government advisory committee suggested that estimated daily energy requirements for adults might be too low, and that people may be able to consume another 400 kcals per day. The newspapers took this and turned it into headlines like 'You can eat an extra cheeseburger a day'. Many of you will hear people on calorie-controlled or points-based diets say things like 'I haven't eaten a thing all day so I can save my points for a massive Chinese takeaway tonight', or 'I'm skipping a meal so I can enjoy a bottle of wine later'. Clearly this is not a sensible approach. With this in mind, if you're not going to suggest just counting calories, then what advice should you give?

- Listen to the body – are clients really hungry? Or are they thirsty, bored, stressed or tired? Read more about this in the food and mood section later in this chapter.

- Create habits – find a routine that works and stick to it as often as possible.
- Monitor progress – use the screening/testing talked about in Chapter 3. If weight/body fat is decreasing then what they're doing is working. If not, review and make changes.
- Identify danger times – it might be Friday night after work with friends, visiting parents or sat at the desk, but work out when someone might overconsume calories and plan ahead.
- Write it down – food diaries, although often inaccurate in terms of exact calories are an effective weight loss tool. This may be because they make people more conscious of what they are eating, or because if they're showing it to someone else, they are less likely to make bad choices for fear of feeling guilty.
- Control portions – find ways to manage the amounts eaten.

Let's have a look at how this could be done.

THANK YOU SIR, I'M FULL NOW AND DON'T NEED ANY MORE

Imagine if this had been the line that Oliver had delivered in the film named after him. It probably wouldn't be as well remembered as it is today. There are a number of ways to control portions without continuously reaching for the calculator. Feel free to use any of the suggestions below, or work with clients to create others that work for them.

PLAN AHEAD

Simply making a shopping list makes a big difference. If people know what they're going for and stick to it, when they look in their cupboards that is all they will find.

Be prepared

Like any good Boy Scout or Girl Guide, encourage clients to be prepared. Suggest making lunch the day before, putting a few handfuls of nuts into some Tupperware instead of taking the entire packet, pouring a few crisps into a small bowl instead of having the whole packet to hand, anything that means they only have what they need. Remember, 'failing to plan is planning to fail'.

Out of sight, out of mind

This old adage can help when it comes to food. Things sat on the kitchen side, or on desks seem to talk to people, usually with a voice similar to that of Gollum in *Lord of the Rings*. 'Go on, you know you wants it, mmmm tastes good in our belly doesn't it?' Silence the gremlins by putting things away.

Size matters

Lots of clients say that eating from smaller plates helps. This is certainly true for couples who eat together; while they will often share the same meal they certainly don't always need the same sized portions, especially if the husband is six foot five and his wife is five foot tall, which I have seen.

The importance of plate size may be related to the Delboeuf illusion, discovered in the nineteenth century by Joseph Delboeuf. It deceives they eye into thinking something is smaller or larger based on the size of the shape that surrounds it. Take a look at the image of the two black circles below.

The black circle on the left appears larger than the one on the right. This is because a larger

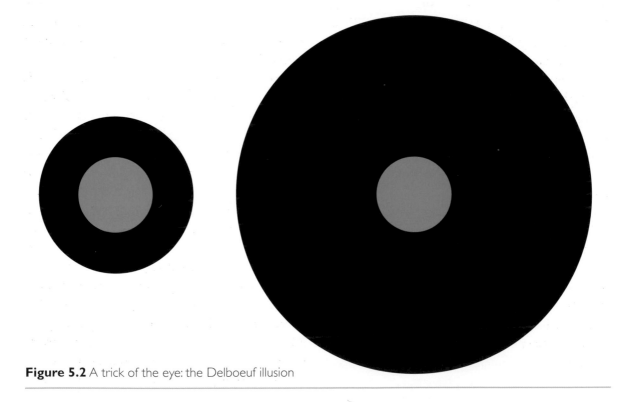

Figure 5.2 A trick of the eye: the Delboeuf illusion

white circle surrounds the one on the right, giving the effect of making it appear proportionately smaller. Now imagine these were plates of food. If someone had the bigger plate they may be tempted to add an extra helping, as it didn't look as filling.

Stop signs

It is not just the size of a plate that can deceive the brain, but also the colour too. Ridiculous, you say? Well, there is science to back this up. It appears that the human brain links the colour red to stopping or danger in many contexts. One report on two studies showed that people ate and drank 40 per cent less when using a red plate and cup when compared to those offered the same portion sizes with blue crockery (Genschow et al, 2012). Yet another study suggested it might be important to contrast the colours of food and plate; they found that people ate more greens if they were served on a green plate, but consumption went down if eaten from a red one (Van Ittersum and Wansink, 2012). This can be used to your advantage in a number of ways:

- If trying to increase vegetable intake, pop them on a plate of the same colour. This may be really helpful for parents encouraging children to eat more.
- If someone wants to decrease the amount of chips they have with their meal, go for something contrasting like a purple plate.

There's no need to insist people go out and buy a rainbow-coloured dinner set for every occasion, but there may be some changes they can try based on this.

Less is, in this case, less.

It has been proposed that if people are given a greater variety of food then they are likely to consume more. This may be because the brain cannot choose between different tastes and so it opts for a bit of everything. This might be a learned behaviour, as it appears that younger children, when given choice, choose what they want, but tend to stop eating earlier, often leaving food on the plate. Many of us when growing up will have been told by family members to 'eat everything on your plate because there are starving children in Africa' or 'you won't be allowed to have any pudding unless you finish your dinner'. The latter basically says that you won't be allowed to eat even more food until you've made yourself full already, which makes no sense at all really.

In today's Western societies, 'all you can eat' buffets are commonplace. Doctors Brian Wansink and Collin Payne (2008) of Cornell University in America studied the eating habits of overweight and normal weight people at Chinese buffets and found that they exhibited quite different behaviours. Those who were heavier chose larger plates, sat closer to the food and often facing it, started to fill their plate before surveying the choices and ate faster, chewing less often. Now these might all be coincidences, or it may be that these habits only come about when someone is already overweight. Nonetheless, if people can become conscious of their eating behaviours they can begin to do something about them. Small changes like choosing only a certain number of foods from a buffet, using smaller plates (we already know this works), or chewing food properly, putting down the knife and fork in between bites, might all be effective. Individuals can try any of these or propose alternatives of their own.

Interestingly, only half as many overweight individuals left food on their plates compared to normal weight diners. Maybe this was learned at childhood dinner tables when their mothers threatened to hold back on the apple pie or chocolate fudge cake?

Chew don't chow

It is often suggested that people should eat slowly as it will ensure that food is broken down and digested more effectively. It is also theorised that eating more slowly means that fullness signals have time to be released, resulting in lower food intake. The scientific literature to back this idea up is pretty thin on the ground, but one study did show that eating slowly could significantly decrease the volume of food consumed and also that people who ate more slowly felt considerably fuller than those who ate faster, even though those who ate more quickly consumed a lot more calories (Andrade et al, 2008). Based on this, it seems it wouldn't do any harm to suggest eating slowly, chewing food properly and putting the knife and fork down in between bites, although there's no conclusive proof that this aids weight loss.

Drink more and weigh less?

An oft-heard notion is that a glass of water before a meal will increase feelings of fullness and decrease the amount of calories consumed. Negoianu and Goldfarb (2008) reviewed the research on this topic and found it to be a mixed bag, providing no conclusive evidence one way or the other. In some instances, drinking water before meals decreased calorie intake during, in others it had no effect. On other occasions drinking water made no difference but adding water to the food itself did decrease calorie intake. At this stage then, it seems that it will not be harmful to drink water with meals but that the claims it will help weight loss cannot be regarded as fact.

QUALITY NOT QUANTITY

Now we've looked at the amount of food to be eaten, let's put the type of grub we consume on the menu. As you've seen, calories and portions should certainly be considered when looking to decrease fat stores, but where those calories come from may be important too. If someone consumed 2,000 grams (500 calories) of broccoli you wouldn't expect it to have the same effect on their body as a 100 gram fruit and nut chocolate bar, which coincidentally also contains 500 calories.

As nutrition is such a large topic, we'll look in turn at each of the different nutrients consumed in the diet. In this context when we talk about 'diet', we'll be referring to the food that people generally consume each day, not an eating pattern that restricts or bans specific foods. This book looks at nutrition purely from a weight loss perspective, as the topic is too vast and worthy of its own book, if not an entire library.

Macronutrients are the major building blocks of any diet and form the largest percentage of what is consumed. These are fats, carbohydrates and proteins.

FAT'S LIFE

Traditionally, when you read books on nutrition, you'll find in most that carbohydrate comes first in any review of macronutrients. As this book deals with the subject of weight loss, and you can't have a conversation about it or see an advert for a food on TV that doesn't mention the fat content of foods, this seemed like a better place to start.

The term fat conjures up images of wobbly bellies, thick pieces of meat, butter and a whole host of foods that supposedly make people pile on the pounds. Derogatory terms used to describe being overweight have close associations with it, including podgy, porky, flabby or lardy. While in the body, excess pounds can and do get stored as fat, it is not the case that all fats make people fat, nor that they are all bad.

Far from it, fat plays an absolutely essential role in the human body for many reasons:

- Vitamins A, D, E and K are fat-soluble. This means they cannot be absorbed without the presence of fat in the diet. These vitamins do all sorts of important things in the body, including maintaining the health and good functioning of hair, skin, bones, teeth, eyes, kidneys, red blood cells, and the ability of blood to clot.
- The brain is made largely of fat. In fact, the entire central nervous system, including the protective layer around the nerves, known as the Myelin Sheath, is composed of fatty acids. It is estimated that two thirds of the brain is fat, yet nobody ever wants to lose a couple of inches off their brain when they join the gym.
- Fats make people happy. Fats are important in the creation of hormones, the substances that perform numerous roles in the body, one of them being to regulate mood.
- Fats offer protection and warmth. A certain amount of fat is needed to provide cushioning and insulation to protect the vital organs.

There are many different types of fat that you can eat. These differ because of their chemical structure and are known as saturated, monoun- saturated, polyunsaturated or hydrogenated – also known as trans-fats.

Saturated fat

You'll all have heard of it and no doubt you'll know that it's found in foods like meat, cheese, butter and milk. You may not, however, know exactly what it is, or be aware of the debate that has been raging around it for the past few years.

Saturated fat is so called because of its chemical structure. All fats have what is known as a carbon chain, a series of carbon atoms linked together, and surrounding these are hydrogen atoms. In saturated fat every carbon atom has two hydrogen atoms surrounding it with no room for any more, hence the term 'saturated'. Why the chemistry lesson you may ask? Well, the chemical structure of a fat affects how it interacts with the human body and it is this that has led to the debate around saturated fat and health.

According to the NHS the current guidelines recommend that men should eat no more than 30 grams per day of saturated fat, while women should only have 20 grams (NHS, 2013). The premise behind this is that higher amounts of saturated fat in the diet increase cholesterol levels in the blood, which in turn increase the risk of heart disease. This has been staple guidance since the 1950s due to research from, among others, a man named Ancel Keys. This has been the cause of great debate since, with some arguing that the original work was flawed due to claims that Keys hand-selected results from countries that supported his theory while leaving out others that did not.

As well as heart disease, consumption of fat with a higher amount of calories per gram has been linked to weight gain. This has led to guid-ance to cut down on saturated fat in order to reduce weight. The problem with this is that fat as a whole has been demonised, leading to the 'lite', 'lighter' and 'low-fat' food culture of today. This may have decreased the intake of harmful fats, but also of essential ones, and at the same time increased the consumption of damaging processed sugars and sweeteners which, it turns out, may have just as much of a role to play in obesity, diabetes and heart disease, if not more.

In recent years there has been a movement by some groups to promote the benefits of saturated fats for health and weight loss. This has included those famous low-carb diet gurus Atkins and Dukan, and even journalists and scientific researchers like Gary Taubes (2008) and Siri-Tarino et al (2010). They argue that there is little hard evidence that it is saturated fat that increases risk of heart disease, certainly in some if not all population groups across the world. Examples often cited are the Inuit tribes of North America and the Masai of Kenya. The low-carb advocates lay the blame for the rise in heart disease and obesity squarely at the feet of highly processed, high-sugar diets. And there is other research that may back up this argument with high-fat diets showing effective weight loss and reduction in insulin levels (Yancy et al, 2004; Samaha et al, 2003).

In 1960s America fat made up around 45 per cent of the diet yet only 13 per cent of the population were obese, with only 1 per cent suffering from type 2 diabetes. Today the average American consumes 33 per cent of their diet as fat, yet 34 per cent of them are obese, and 11 per cent have type 2 diabetes. Even this is the subject of debate, with the US Department for Agriculture (USDA, 1998) reporting that total calorie consumption has increased in America over the past 30 years, and that people are taking on substantially more calories. These are coming largely from processed carbohydrates like biscuits, white pasta and fizzy drinks, which is why the overall percentage of calories from fat has gone down. The USDA does, however, suggest that the actual amount of fat consumed has increased, it's just that carbohydrate consumption has increased more, sending the percentage of the total diet down.

Even one of the UK's senior surgeons has waded into the argument. Dr Aseem Malhotra has spoken out to say that he believes more attention should be placed on reducing sugar intake and encouraging a diet high in fruit, vegetables and oily fish (BBC News, 2013).

While the debate is as yet unresolved, it seems prudent to say that if saturated fats are to be consumed, they should come from natural produce such as butter, cheese, milk and meat. Portion size should be considered, as calorie consumption still needs to be factored in. Processed foods high in saturated fat, trans-fats and sugar should be limited.

Unsaturated fats

Monounsaturated and polyunsaturated fats are so called because of their respective biochemical structures. Monounsaturated fats have one hydrogen atom missing from the carbon chain and have a double bond between the associated carbons. Polyunsaturated fats have at least two double bonds.

Both have been reported to improve cholesterol levels, and as such from a health perspective are considered good fats by many. Unsaturated fats come from nuts and seeds, oily fish and some fruit and vegetables including avocados, which are a particularly rich source.

Omega 3: It's mega!

Of all the unsaturated fats, Omega 3, a particular type of polyunsaturated fat, has been shown to be most important for health, hence it being referred to as an 'essential fat'. Omega 3 intake in the UK is lower than it should be for health, while intakes of Omega 6 and 9 are reportedly too high. Work with clients to increase their intake of oily fish and avocado and encourage clients to get smaller amounts of 6 and 9 from plant-based foods. This may help to:

- Decrease blood pressure
- Decrease risk of heart arrhythmias
- Decrease risk of coronary artery disease
- Decrease cancer risk in some
- Improve mood and decrease instances of depression

Parra et al (2008) suggest that Omega 3 may even increase feelings of fullness after a meal, and with all of this evidence it's important to encourage a good intake of oily fish. Current recommendations are for a minimum of one portion per week, but in reality two–four portions would be better. Many people don't enjoy consuming oily fish so a way round this is to mix it into recipes. Examples include: fish pie made with salmon and white fish. The latter is lower in Omega 3 but salmon contains good amounts. Stirring mackerel into a paella containing strong flavours like chorizo can make it more palatable for some too. It should be remembered that while fresh tuna is rich in Omega 3, tinned tuna generally contains lower levels, equivalent to white fish.

Trans-fatty acids

Cue the pantomime villains. The vast majority of trans-fatty acids, also called trans-fats, hydrogenated or partially hydrogenated fats, have been shown to be bad for health, increasing the risk of diabetes, heart disease and possibly other conditions too.

What are trans-fats? They are fats that have been 'twisted' and this change in their structure allows them to preserve the shelf life of the foods they are found within, commonly pastries, biscuits, cakes and other processed goodies, or in this case 'baddies'.

It is recommended that trans-fats should make up less than 2 per cent of total diet, and since restrictions have been put in place on their use in foods, this has generally been shown to be the case. For individuals still consuming large amounts of processed or convenience foods, encourage them to decrease these to lower their trans-fat intake.

CARBOHYDRATES

In recent years carbohydrates have had a pretty hard time, battered by the numerous low-carb diets and demonised for making us fat and causing diabetes. Like all things in nutrition, it's never quite that simple. There are different types of carbohydrates and the many varied foods within this group can have wildly varying effects on the body.

Firstly, again let's start by saying that carbohydrates play some essential roles. Many will argue that they're the preferred source of energy for the body; they're certainly the quickest to break down. They also play a key part in fat metabolism, breaking it down fully to be used as energy. Finally, the brain relies on a steady supply of sugar from the blood to keep it functioning.

Everyone has experienced that feeling of fuzziness and confusion brought about by slightly low blood sugars. Those of you who exercise regularly may even have 'hit the wall' as they say in running circles, or 'bonked' as those who prefer the bicycle call it, when blood sugars drop to a level that causes performance to plummet.

Carbohydrates clearly have a role to play, but again it comes down to type, how much and when they are consumed, and a person's individual needs and responses. Too much carbohydrate, in particular refined sugars, appear to be as bad as too much fat, sending blood sugar levels soaring and leading to weight gain and type 2 diabetes if eaten too often. If the body's stores of carbohydrate (glycogen in muscles and the liver) are already topped up to the maximum, then any excess can be converted to fat and stored away. Worse still, sugars send insulin levels up rapidly and insulin is, as you know, the hormone that promotes the storage of energy in the body. Combine this with the fact that many foods high in refined sugars are also high in trans- and saturated fats then it really is a recipe for disaster.

The original focus on carbohydrates was whether they were complex or simple. This wasn't to do with the nature of their character; instead it referred to their structure. Complex carbohydrates are made up of three or more sugars in chains, whereas simple carbohydrates have just one or two. Complex carbohydrates are referred to as starches, or cellulose, and are found in wholegrain produce, vegetables and legumes. Simple carbohydrates include glucose, lactose (milk sugar) and fructose (fruit sugar). It was generally considered that complex carbohydrates were better as they broke down more slowly, but in recent years a more useful classification of carbs has emerged: the glycaemic index.

GLYCAEMIC INDEX

The glycaemic index, or GI, identifies the speed at which sugar is broken down in the bloodstream. The more quickly this happens, the higher the GI of the food, with foods generally being classified as low, medium or high GI. Each food is scored out of 100, showing how quickly it elevates blood sugars in comparison to pure table sugar. The higher the GI score, the quicker the release of sugar into the bloodstream. Scores are classified as shown in Figure 5.3.

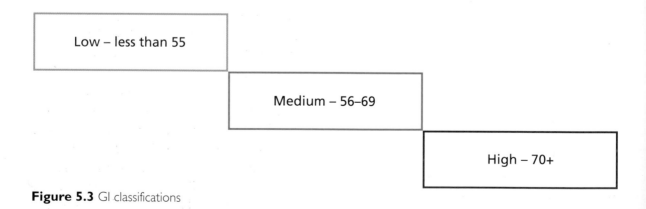

Low – less than 55

Medium – 56–69

High – 70+

Figure 5.3 GI classifications

Other than immediately before, or during sports events, high GI foods are not a good thing. Twenty miles into a marathon, people need a sugar hit to keep them going so high GI foods are the way to go, but sat at a desk or in the car, high GI foods offer no benefits.

When high GI foods are consumed, blood sugar levels rise quickly. The body responds by releasing insulin from the pancreas, returning blood sugar levels to normal and storing away lots of energy in the process. If the two places that need stored carbohydrate are full (the liver and the muscles) then it moves to plan B. This involves the conversion of carbohydrate into fat, to be stored away as adipose tissue. The body does this because, not that long ago in the grand scheme of things, human beings had to fight for survival in a harsh environment. Food could be scarce and so any opportunity to save energy was extremely helpful from an evolutionary standpoint. Unfortunately, evolution at a genetic level takes thousands of years, and

in a very short space of time Western civilisation has developed a whole host of things to make life easier. These include processed foods, the car and the supermarket. As opposed to having to go out hunting or scavenging for food for a number of hours, then gather it, catch it, carry it home and prepare it, we now put our coats on, pick up the car keys, drive to the local store, put a few items in a trolley, put it in the boot, get home, press a few buttons on a microwave and consume. This clearly doesn't require the same amount of energy, and there's no real necessity to store energy away in our bodies any more, we can do that in the cupboard, freezer or, if we really have to, we can drive back to the shop, a real inconvenience of course but it is just about manageable. The more tech-savvy may just put an online order in, save themselves the effort and ensure they don't miss *X Factor*.

With our evolutionary make-up in mind, it can be extremely useful to understand the GI of different foods, and to consume low GI options the majority of the time. There are plenty of online resources that reveal the GI of thousands of foods, but below are some useful guidelines, and Table 5.2 outlines some foods that fall under the low, medium and high categories.

- Is it processed? If a food is in its natural state, it tends to have a lower GI than if it has been altered. See the information on fruit juice later as an example.
- How fresh is it? In relation to fruits and vegetables, the less ripe the produce the lower the GI. A green banana for example, is less broken down that a soft one with all of its distinctive brown spots. The speckled one has its sugars more readily available and as such will be released more quickly into the bloodstream.

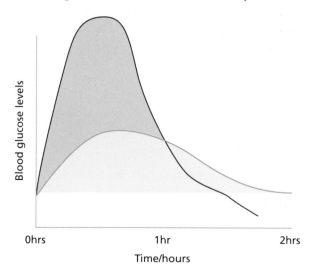

Figure 5.4 The blood sugar rollercoaster: responses to high and low GI foods

- Don't stress too much about fruit and vegetables. If they're in their natural state they've got plenty of good things in them too. Eat a mixture and try to have slightly more vegetables than fruit.
- Food combining affects GI. Few people eat one food on its own; generally it forms part of a meal. If a high GI food is combined with a low one, then the overall GI of the meal is moderated (see more on this in the glycaemic load section). As an example, baked potatoes tend to have a high GI, but they are often consumed with chicken, butter, tuna or other higher fat, higher protein foods that tend to have very low, or even no GI. Foods without carbohydrates present do not have a GI, as they don't affect blood sugar levels.
- Cooking increases GI. This doesn't mean that foods shouldn't be cooked; it's just something to be aware of. As mentioned above, a baked potato for example, generally has a high GI, whereas when raw, a potato's GI is lower. Obviously this doesn't mean that potatoes should be the next cold snack, there'd be a few teeth lost this way, but it should serve to make people aware about cooking. Roast parsnips

Table 5.2	The GIs of foods commonly consumed in the UK	
Low GI	**Medium GI**	**High GI**
Carrots (raw)	Most cooked pasta	Watermelon
Apples	Peaches	Scones
Pears	Wholemeal pitta bread	White bread, bagel or baguette
Oranges	Raisins/sultanas	Energy drinks (Gatorade, Lucozade)
Dark chocolate (generally 70% cocoa solids or more)	Peaches	Watermelon
Milk	Wholemeal pitta bread	Scones
Wholegrain rice	Bananas	Doughnuts
Wild rice	Couscous	Cornflakes and many other breakfast cereals
Custard		
Lentils		
Natural yoghurt		

and roast potatoes for example, have higher GIs than steamed parsnips and lightly boiled spuds, so a few changes to the Sunday roast can be effective.

- All foods are not equal. Everything that goes into a food affects its GI and foods that you would think would be quite similar, can have large differences in GI. To take an example, a popular chocolate bar that was once reported to help you work, rest and play (its sugar content is certainly unlikely to make the first two true) has a fairly high GI (in the 60s), whereas its competitor, famed for its mix of chocolate and peanuts comes in much lower, generally around 40, due to its higher nut content. This is where common sense comes in to play, regularly consuming low GI chocolate bars won't help weight loss or health, but making sensible choices when consuming one occasionally, coupled with a healthy diet packed full of unprocessed foods, will.

The GI of a given food can vary hugely. This can be down to how it is grown or processed, where in the world it comes from, how long after picking, making or cooking it is tested and, of course, the science behind the testing process. In fact, many foods can vary greatly in the score given depending on which GI study is used. Rye bread can be anywhere from low to high depending on whether it is mixed with other flours or substances. Pineapple in its purest form may be low, but tinned it could well be high. Sweet potato, while low in its raw state, is obviously eaten cooked and can be medium or even high depending on whether it is baked, roasted or mashed and how long it is cooked for. GI is a guide, one piece of useful information

Juicing your way to five a day?

It is pretty common these days to see adverts for healthy fruit juice drinks or to find an aisle full of them in the shops. But recent research suggests that they may not be as good as they are made out to be. The research appears pretty unequivocal – regular consumption of fruit juice increases the risk for type 2 diabetes and weight gain. A recent study across a number of countries showed that drinking fruit juice increased the risk of developing these conditions, but eating fruit decreased it. When people swapped from juice to real fruit, their risk of illness decreased by 7 per cent. This may well be because the fructose intake with fruit juice is much more concentrated than it is when consumed as fruit. Juicing breaks down the fibre in fruit and may well increase the GI (Boseley, 2013).

It is healthier and may be more effective for weight loss to consume real fruit and to opt for vegetable juices if juicing at all.

for healthy eating, but not the be-all and end-all. In many cases, the less processed the food the lower the GI.

GLYCAEMIC LOAD

Glycaemic load, or GL, is a useful addition to the research in this area. GI only measures the rate of sugar released in a fixed amount of a food, normally 50 grams. It does not take into account how much carbohydrate is in an actual serving of a food, and as such can sometimes be misleading. An example is watermelon; it has a high GI but, as you can tell by its name, is largely made up of water. Therefore, although its sugars release very quickly into the bloodstream, because it does not contain that much, the effect on the body's blood sugar levels is minimal. A chocolate bar however, has a high GI and also a high content of carbohydrate and therefore a high GL.

It is calculated as follows:

$$GI \times \text{carbohydrate in food (grams)} \div 100$$

So for example, if a white bagel contained 30 grams of carbohydrate and had a GI of 75, it would have the following GL:

$$30 \times 75 = 2,250 \div 100 = 22.5$$

This would put a white bagel in the high category based on the norm's values for GL, which are:

Low – less than 10
Medium – 11–19
High – 20+

So if the GI of the food is known, the GL can be calculated based on the size of the serving consumed. Even without weighing or calculating anything the message is clear: if eating high GI foods, combine them with low GI or no GI ones to bring down the overall GL of the meal or snack. Examples could be:

- Jacket potato with butter, chicken, tuna, mackerel, cottage cheese or beans
- Chicken, turkey, beef or other meat sandwiches
- Banana with a handful of nuts
- Couscous with fish

WHAT DOES THE SCIENCE SAY?

Regular consumption of high GI foods leads to weight gain and increased body fat, as well as increased risk of type 2 diabetes. In a review of numerous studies on appetite and GI, all but one showed that the lower the GI of a food, the longer an individual would be satiated (full up) (Ludwig, 2000). The same review also found that eating higher GI foods consistently stimulated insulin release in both human and animal tests, and that this led to increased hunger and fat storage, making weight gain likely. It also concluded that when people opted for low-fat diets, as often advised, the GI of their meals went up considerably.

Figure 5.5 shows examples of foods that should be consumed and those that should be limited as part of a low GI diet.

FIBRE FOR FAT LOSS?

Fibre, sometimes referred to as roughage, is a type of carbohydrate found predominantly in plant foods. It has achieved attention for its potential to assist weight loss and digestive health, although as is the usual for nutrition, there are conflicting views. There are two types of fibre and dependent on type, they may have a number of health benefits:

- Soluble fibre – this can be digested and may decrease cholesterol levels, prevent constipation and type 2 diabetes.
- Insoluble fibre – this cannot be digested by the body and may possibly reduce risk of bowel cancer and type 2 diabetes.

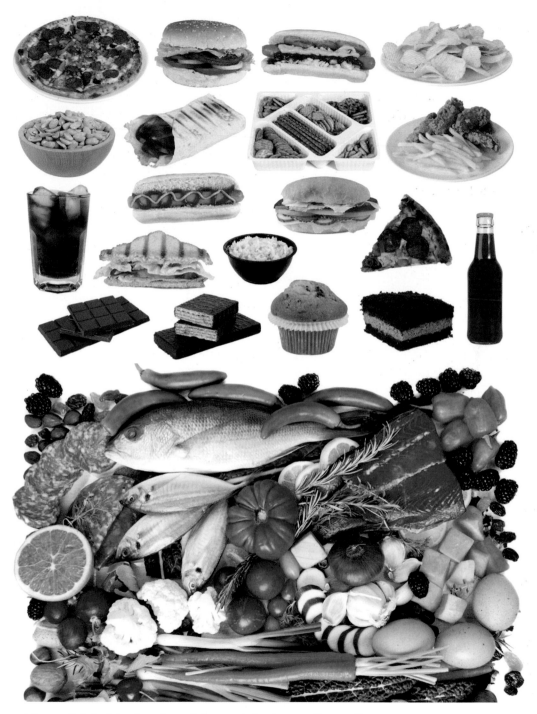

Figure 5.5 Bad (top) and good (bottom) foods according to GI

Table 5.3	Sources of soluble and insoluble fibre	
Soluble	**Insoluble**	
• Fruit and vegetables	• Cereals and bran	
• Legumes, lentils, pulses and beans	• Nuts and seeds	
• Oats, barley and rye	• Wholemeal bread	
• Golden linseed	• Wholemeal pasta and wholegrain rice	
	• Fruit and vegetables	

What about weight loss? Well, a healthy digestive system is a good start so it may have a role to play there. It has also been shown, like protein, to increase feelings of fullness possibly by reducing the amount people eat. Fibre has long been seen as a 'free' food, filling but containing no calories, and while this is true for a lot of fibre, some does contain energy. Recently it has been claimed that high-fibre foods may have been misleading people for a number of years by not showing the calories contained within them on the label, with maybe as much as 5 per cent of energy in a food coming from fibre (Connor, 2013).

Even so it may well have a role to play in weight loss. This is due to its filling effect, absorbing water and sitting in the stomach for longer, plus the fact that it takes longer to chew and break down, allowing the body and brain to release signals to say it is full. The famous diet spawned from this, the F-Plan, may have worked however because it advocated a low-calorie lifestyle, returning once again to the common theme across all diets: portion control.

The pro-high-protein camp may not advocate higher fibre diets, largely because of the fact that much of it is found in wheat. Obviously for those who are wheat allergic, and for those with conditions such as IBS, adaptations need to be made. It is still possible to consume fibre without the need for wholemeal bread and pasta, opting instead for small amounts of fruit, vegetables, wholegrain rice, nuts, seeds, pulses, beans and lentils. Those with IBS should work with a dietician and be guided by their symptoms.

PROTEIN GETS YOU LEAN?

Protein, made up of amino acids, has an important role in making enzymes and hormones, blood clotting, fighting infection by building antibodies, and also for making most of the tissues in the body, including hair, skin, bone and muscle. When most people think of dietary protein, they think of it as something bodybuilders eat to get big muscles. This has an element of truth to it, but it's a vital nutrient for everyone to help maintain muscle tissue, or lean mass as it is sometimes known. It isn't just for those who want to look like Arnie in his heyday; it's for everyone. As you saw earlier in the book, muscle mass helps to maintain metabolic activity. It is also clear that as people age they lose muscle mass (Sreekumaran Nair, 2005). This starts in the 30s and may be a key reason as to why it becomes harder over time to keep body fat levels down.

Obviously to keep lean mass people need to exercise, but they also need to eat adequate protein. The amount needed, however, is under debate. The current recommendation for protein consumption is around 10–15 per cent of total diet (British Nutrition Foundation, 2012); however, most people consume more than this already. Some argue that high-protein diets (greater than

25 per cent) are the best way to lose weight and be healthy, and diet creators, including Atkins and Dukan among others, have championed this.

WHAT DOES THE SCIENCE SAY?

High-protein diets can work for weight loss; replacement of carbohydrate with protein has been shown to lead to weight loss and health benefits in obese people and for those with diabetes (Skov et al, 1999; Noakes et al, 2005; Parker et al, 2002). Some studies in this area should be treated with caution as they were funded by the very organisations that promote high-protein diets, but this does not mean they are not valid. Further research has been carried out independently and still shown effective weight loss. There are inconsistencies, however, with other studies showing no benefits. Astrup, Larsen and Harper (2004) and Halton and Hu (2004) suggest that calorie intake is key and that both high-protein and high-carbohydrate diets can result in weight loss.

Some high-protein diets show improvements in other health and weight loss markers when compared to higher carbohydrate intake. These include:

- Higher satiation after meals, leading to decreased eating afterwards.
- Increased dietary thermogenesis. This is the increase in calorie burn resulting from the effort needed to digest food.
- Improved insulin sensitivity.

Are there any potential downsides to high-protein diets? Possibly. High-protein diets may lead to high fat intake as many foods contain both. It should also be remembered that excess calories, even if they come from protein are converted into and stored as fat. Many assume that this is only true of carbohydrates and fats but energy is energy, regardless of where it comes from and if stores are full the body will find a way to keep hold of it.

Two key concerns have been raised in the scientific community about high-protein diets. The first relates to kidney function. High protein consumption (diets containing more than 25–30 per cent protein) lead to *ketosis*, when acidic compounds known as ketones are made in the body. It occurs because adequate carbohydrate is needed to break down fats completely. With low-carb diets, fat breaks down partially and ketones are produced. As a response to ketone build-up, the kidneys have to work harder to remove them. They are flushed out with water when urinating and dehydration can occur. Dehydration can in turn put more strain on the kidneys, creating a vicious circle. One common sign of ketosis is bad breath, some will say that it smells like pear drops or nail varnish due to its high acid content, but others will tell you that it has an even less pleasant odour.

The science world is still debating if this poses an issue, partly because there is sometimes disagreement as to what constitutes a 'high-protein' diet, with some saying 30 per cent while others arguing that it may be as much as 50 per cent. On top of this, the effects of these diets may differ greatly between athletes, overweight individuals and those with recognised medical conditions. At present it is agreed that those with current kidney conditions should not consume high-protein diets (Friedman, 2004), and diabetics should also be very cautious, only altering their diet after consulting their medical practitioner (Eisenstein et al, 2002).

The other major concern is risk for osteoporosis. Protein rich foods are acidic as they are made up of amino acids, high-protein diets are therefore acidic. Bones have been shown to assist the kidneys in controlling higher levels of acid in the blood – calcium can leach from bones into the bloodstream, making it more alkaline and bringing it back into balance. Unfortunately, if this occurs for long periods, calcium levels in bones may fall. Even six weeks on a high-protein diet is long enough for blood acid levels to rise, increasing the risk for bone mass loss and kidney stone formation (Reddy et al, 2002).

WATER AND WEIGHT

Finally, an area of nutrition where science can agree on something: what is it, you wonder? It's water, and it's good for you. OK, so there's still plenty of debate as to exactly what it does, how much should be consumed and a host of other questions, but hey, it's a start.

Between half and three quarters of the body is water, the blood consists of more than 80 per cent of the stuff, and it's a major part of every single cell, so it's no wonder that it's important to keep well hydrated. There has been a lot of research on the effects of water on performance. It's known that dehydration will decrease endurance by as much as 10 per cent, strength by 2 per cent, power by 3 per cent and can even affect motor skills (Judelson et al, 2007).

Even the diet books agree that water is good, with everything from Atkins to The Zone Diet recommending an intake of around 1.5–2 litres per day. This makes sense if you think about it, a car wouldn't perform optimally without being topped up with fluid, so why should the body?

The problem has always been that, while it seems fairly obvious that drinking enough is important, the scientific literature on the effects of water outside of sports is sparse, or to put it another way, the well is empty.

OLD WIVES' TALES OF WATER

Table 5.4 lists some 'facts' you'll hear about water and lets you know just how much evidence there is to support them.

There's some evidence then that water helps weight loss, and a little to suggest that drinking enough helps maintain health. Certainly not drinking any leads to death in a matter of days, so it makes sense that smaller amounts of dehydration would be detrimental to a lesser degree. Below are some guidelines to use for water consumption:

- Follow the recommended guidelines and aim to drink between 1.5–2 litres per day.
- The amount of fluid consumed may need to increase if exercising. The American College of Sports Medicine recommends 3–8 ounces (75–225 millilitres) of water every 15–20 minutes for up to an hour. After this point the same fluid is recommended but sugary drinks will be needed as the body's energy stores run low. This means about three to four glasses of water, or just under a litre, every hour (ACSM, 2011).
- In reality people may not have to drink this much, as food contains water too. Fruit and vegetables are particularly rich in fluids and help towards fluid needs.
- Consider the calories – sugary, fizzy drinks containing corn syrup, and even diet drinks containing sweeteners, are now shown to increase the risk for weight gain and diabetes.

Table 5.4	Water: truth or myth?
Water 'fact'	**Truth or myth?**
Being dehydrated increases blood pressure	As it stands there is little scientific backing for this claim.
Dehydration is linked to blood sugar imbalances	Dehydration certainly has been linked to fatigue, but at present there is little evidence in healthy populations to show this is down to changes in blood sugar levels. In diabetics there is a clear link between dehydration and blood glucose, with dehydration occurring if blood sugars get too high. This happens in diabetics as the body deals with excessively high glucose levels by flushing it out in urine. Going to the toilet frequently causes dehydration and thirst, common symptoms used to diagnose the condition.
Dehydration decreases mental performance and mood	Mental performance does decrease with mild dehydration.
Dehydration causes headaches	There is strangely little research on this. However, one recent study asked people to record whether or not they had headaches when they were dehydrated. The results indicated that this was common and that headaches would go away quickly if water were consumed. They also noted that there were numerous references on the Internet to people who stated that dehydration brought about migraines (Blau, 2004).
Drinking water regularly helps weight loss	There is little research out there to back up this statement. One or two studies have shown that increased water consumption may improve the amount of weight lost. In one study water was given to participants in the half hour before meals, resulting in 13 per cent less calories consumed (Davy et al, 2008). Another looked at women on various different diets and while the aim was to compare the effectiveness of each diet, they noticed a secondary effect, namely that higher water intake was associated with greater success in weight loss across all diets over time (Stookey et al, 2008). Other studies have shown little effect.
Tea and coffee dehydrate you	Tea and coffee, although containing caffeine, will not dehydrate, as the largest proportion of what's in the cup is water. Herbal tea, milk and diluted squash/fruit juice will hydrate although pure fruit juice may not do so effectively as its high sugar content slows down the rate of absorption.

FOOD FOR THOUGHT

Cutting these out or limiting them is a very effective tool for weight loss. Pure fruit juice, as already mentioned earlier in the chapter, increases risk for diabetes because of its high fructose concentration.

- Drink water before eating. One or two glasses before food may fill the stomach and decrease calorie intake. Certainly swapping sugary drinks for water will lessen calorie intake dramatically.
- Limit alcohol – more on this in Chapter 7, but again, there's a lot of calories and not much goodness going on, especially if drinking more than one or two glasses.
- Bottle it. Carrying a water bottle around can substantially increase fluid intake as it acts as a reminder to drink.
- Take the pee test. The colour of urine is an excellent marker of levels of hydration; light, straw coloured urine suggests good hydration but if it is dark, more fluids are needed.

MICRONUTRIENTS, BUT MASSIVELY IMPORTANT

From a health perspective, the benefits of vitamins, minerals, antioxidants, flavonoids, polyphenols and other compounds is unquestionable. But do they have any role to play in losing weight or keeping it off? To say yes conclusively would be to stand on very shaky ground, but this doesn't mean they're not important.

Vitamins, minerals and all the other members of our personal health army perform innumerable vital tasks in making the body function correctly. This includes energy production, metabolism of nutrients, muscle growth and repair, cell growth, immune function, blood sugar regulation, bone regeneration and a million other things. Because of this it would be wrong to say that micronutrients don't play a part in weight loss, it's just probably not as clear-cut as some would wish. Taking a pill that contains high levels of one single vitamin may not make a big difference, whereas ensuring adequate intake of a range of micronutrients can help keep the body functioning correctly and maintain health.

Research has provided clear links between a lack of micronutrients in the diet and diseases such as cancer, diabetes, heart disease and osteoporosis. This is in stark contrast to the vitamin and mineral deficiency diseases of times gone by, such as scurvy or rickets that are now very rare in Western society (Fletcher and Fairfield, 2002).

One nutrient that may impact weight is chromium. This mineral appears to play a very important part in blood sugar regulation. In its most readily available form in the body, Chromium picolinate, it has been shown in various studies to:

- Improve insulin sensitivity in those with a family history of diabetes.
- Reduce the insulin dosage needed in type 1 diabetics.
- Consistently benefit those with type 2 diabetes, lowering insulin levels, improving symptoms of the condition and also decreasing blood sugar levels after meals (Anderson, 2000).

The amount taken varies across the studies but the recommended guideline is 200 micrograms per day, with higher intake appearing safe (Anderson, 2000). Chromium is found in broccoli, cheese, turkey, chicken, wholegrains, black pepper, thyme, eggs, corn on the cob, sweet potatoes, grape juice and brewer's yeast, a fungus used in making beer and sold as a supplement.

Regardless of the benefits of certain individual nutrients, getting a balanced diet remains the best place to start. General advice to ensure adequate consumption of micronutrients includes:

- Eat a mixture of different coloured fruit and vegetables, and vary what is consumed to ensure a wide variety of different vitamins, minerals and antioxidants.
- Consume a mixture of nuts, seeds, beans, pulses and lentils in the diet.
- Go grass-fed for meat, butter, and milk, and use free-range organic eggs. Remember that animals eat plants and therefore absorb nutrients too. In theory, the healthier the animal, the more they'll pass on.
- It may not hurt to take a multivitamin/multimineral with antioxidants. Lots of big brands sell these nowadays but people should check with their GP if taking any medications or if they have medical conditions.

MEAL TIMING

Of all the information about when to eat, the advice to *always eat breakfast* has the most evidence to back it up. If the first meal of the day is missed then it is far more likely that poor food choices will be made later on. A healthy breakfast like porridge or eggs can start the day off right, maintain energy levels, balance blood sugars and regulate mood to help face the challenges ahead.

There is less evidence to support the notion that eating 'small and often' is any better than using standard meal times, but advising people not to skip meals and to stick to a routine helps ensure that excessive hunger does not lead to poor food choices. Ever been hungry and noticed that the cake in the shop looks a lot more tempting than usual?

BAD FOOD AND FAKE FOOD

Hopefully it is now clear what foods may be useful, but what about what not to eat, or certainly what to limit? There are a number of things in this category to achieve successful fat loss and weight maintenance. Foods to limit include:

- Processed/refined sugars such as corn syrup
- Sugary or sweetened drinks
- Trans-fats
- Heavily processed foods (generally containing all of the above)
- Alcohol (covered in detail in Chapter 7)

Whether or not these foodstuffs are limited or removed completely is down to the individual, their needs, and how they prefer to achieve their goals in a way that is sustainable. For many the thought of cutting out foods completely seems too hard and can lead to cravings and epic falls from grace where all the good work of a few weeks can be undone in a single evening. For others, abstinence is the best way as they find it difficult to have 'just one piece' or 'only a handful' of whatever their weakness is.

WHY SHOULD THESE THINGS BE LIMITED?

Processed sugar causes a steep rise in insulin, the master hormone for storing energy away. Many processed foods with high levels of refined sugar often also contain high levels of trans-fats or saturated fats as well. Eaten together this can provide the perfect environment for fat storage, as insulin draws all of that energy into those eagerly waiting adipocytes (fat cells).

As you've seen with drinks, they can have a big impact on insulin levels and it appears that the body fails to register the calories from liquids in quite the same way as it does calories from food (Apovian, 2004). This may have something to do with the fact that the stomach is not filled when drinking calories.

Of course, most people know a lot of this already and are probably disappointed that there isn't some radical 'wonder food' that sucks up fat and removes it instantly from the body. The challenge lies in overcoming the urges to eat bad foods caused by a host of physiological and emotional drivers, in a world where so many things have come together to promote convenience, lack of movement and cheap, readily available, low-quality 'food'. To overcome this takes:

- A plan – much like exercise needs a programme, an eating strategy is essential. Creating shopping lists, planning the week's meals, preparing food to take to work all mean the choices available will be healthy ones.
- Support – as per the planning section earlier in the book, key family members and friends need to help out.
- A 'cheat day' or treat schedule – many people find it works to plan a few little treats across the week. It is fairly normal for bodybuilders to schedule a treat day once a week and the same technique can be applied for those trying to lose weight. Really the only difference between bodybuilders and those trying to lose weight

is the amount of muscle they have, both want low amounts of body fat. It doesn't even have to be a cheat day, it can just be scheduled times for treats. Some may choose a certain amount of treats to have in a week and tick them off in a food diary as they have them. Many will talk about the 80:20 rule, eating well 80 per cent of the time and not so healthily for the other 20 per cent.

- Belief and resilience – often it is the importance of the goal to the individual that determines how much effort someone will put into their weight loss programme. If goals are personal to them, SMART and regularly reviewed then this can keep someone focused. With dietary changes, it is highly unlikely that people will always eat perfectly – we need to eat too often, and life is too busy and varied these days for things not to go wrong occasionally. The challenge comes when things do go wrong; do they forget about having a weak moment and start to eat healthily again or do they feel down and spiral into days or weeks of poor eating until they decide they want to do something about it again? In reality the former is the only logical choice if success is desired.

Unhealthy, processed food is calorie dense with little nutritional value. This means that there are lots of calories in very small portions and as such portion control with these 'foods' is considerably more important than controlling the amount of broccoli or carrots consumed. This is important as because processed foods are not particularly filling it can be very easy to eat a large amount of calories quickly and not feel full. Separating out chocolates, biscuits and sweets into smaller portions by using Tupperware or bowls may be a good idea. Putting the rest away out of sight can also help to prevent the temptation to go back for more. Opt for smaller pizzas, cut cake into more pieces, use smaller plates and smaller glasses for drinks and treats can still be enjoyed without preventing goals from being achieved.

FOOD AND MOOD

It is now well established that the brain and the mouth are linked by more than the fact that they both live within a few inches of each other. How a person feels has a major impact on the food choices they make, and in turn what goes into the body can affect hormone levels and change mood states (Ottley, 2000; Appleton and Rogers, 2004; Beimers, 2012).

Various mood states can influence food choice, both positively and negatively. This may be because feelings are often associated with certain actions, known in the world of neurolinguistic programming as anchors. It is also likely that it is down to the fact that some junk foods can alter levels of hormones, temporarily increasing positive feelings. When feeling low, many may use them as a crutch to boost their mood.

There are a huge number of mood states that can impact eating behaviours, and in recent years a number of people have written specifically about this as a means of weight loss as opposed to focusing on the actual foods consumed (McKenna, 2005; Peer, 2008).

As can be seen, there are a wide range of moods that can change eating patterns and these can be influenced by deep-seated subconscious behaviours stemming back to childhood. Many people can address these with their fitness instructor or personal trainer and plan ways to manage their eating during the danger times but others who have a more serious problem with food that may pose

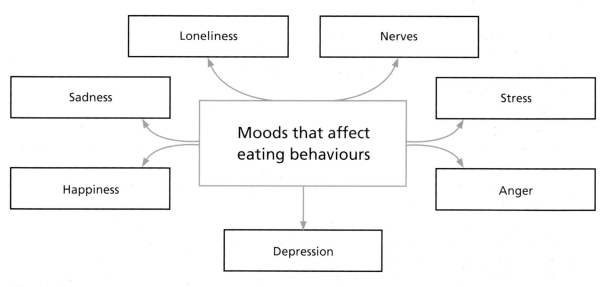

Figure 5.6 Moods that affect eating behaviours

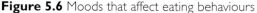

a risk to their health or wellbeing should consult with a GP or qualified counsellor. See more about counselling for weight loss in Chapter 8.

ENVIRONMENTAL FACTORS

This doesn't mean that the amount of sunshine or rainfall causes weight gain, although weather can have a huge impact on mood, with sunlight increasing 'feel good' hormones and cold, dark winters being closely linked with decreases in mood, known commonly as Seasonal Affective Disorder, or SAD. Bear in mind though, there are overweight people in sunny countries too.

In this case the environment relates to situational factors or times when eating habits are worse. This might be a trip to the parents' house or to see the in-laws, Friday night in the pub with friends or colleagues, a trip to the cinema with the oh so tempting pic' 'n' mix options, birthdays, weddings or any other time that acts as a trigger to an individual.

Life stages can be particularly important for nutritional changes. Going to university, leaving home, getting promoted, entering a relationship, the menopause and others can all have a major impact on eating choices and as such these need to be considered and action plans put into place. Youngsters may not have the same level of control over this as their parents, carers or educational environment may largely decide what they eat. That is why Jamie Oliver, to his credit, has campaigned so hard to change what is served in the school canteen and no doubt this will have a significant impact over time. Going to university or leaving home are particularly risky times; often when income is low and there is a fun world out there to be explored, what gets bought at the shops may not be the highest quality, and a diet of instant noodles, crisps, chocolate and fizzy drinks is not uncommon.

PLATES, PYRAMIDS, PERCENTAGES AND PREFERENCES

This chapter has shown that with food, both the quality and quantity have a role to play in successful weight loss. Government agencies have spent a lot of time and money on developing a range of charts, diagrams and guidelines to help people make healthier decisions. These have been changed a number of times over the years and have always been greeted with a mixture of praise and derision from various parties.

The following are, or have been, used by governments in Western society to offer advice on how much of any given food should be consumed:

- RDAs, RDIs, DRVs, RNIs and EARs – these stand for 'recommended daily allowance', 'recommended daily intake', 'dietary reference values', 'reference nutrient intakes' and 'estimated average requirements', and in various ways describe the amounts that people should consume of different nutrients, including carbohydrates, fats, protein, vitamins and minerals.
- Percentages – particularly used for macronutrients, agencies have often recommended how much of any one food type people should eat as a percentage of their overall diet. Present government guidelines around the world generally have starchy, non-refined carbohydrate at around 50–60 per cent of the diet, fat at no more than 35 per cent with around 10 per cent coming from saturated fat, and 10–15

per cent from protein. As you've seen these percentages are points of contention.

- Pyramids – no the ancient Egyptians haven't been involved in directing government policy on food. In the 1980s the first food pyramid appeared in an attempt to show people visually what their diet should look like overall. As a visual it was easily memorable but it didn't really bear any relation to how people went about buying or preparing food.

  In the 2000s the United States Department for Agriculture updated the pyramid, drawing it in vertical lines as opposed to the original boxed approach. It also usefully included exercises on the side of the pyramid, referencing the impor-

tance of daily exercise and activity. The visual was still confusing but the mypyramid.gov website did allow individuals to build their own version that worked for them. The pyramids were based on a high carbohydrate diet.

- Plates – in recent years in both the USA and the UK, they have adopted choosemyplate.gov (USDA, 2013) and the eatwell plate (Crown Copyright, 2013) as their visual eating guides. Plates are arguably a more logical way to go in terms of guides, as it is what many people eat their food from, you don't see many carrying pyramid-shaped Tupperware around with them. Interestingly, while the percentage guidelines have not changed, both plates do

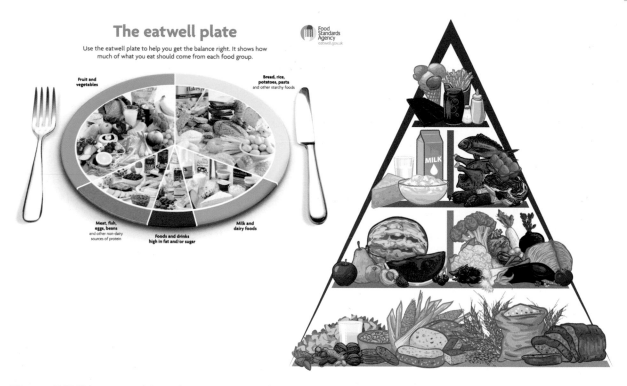

Figure 5.7 Plates, pyramids and percentages: various ways to represent ideal food intake

show a small swing in favour of consuming more vegetables than grains, with the area for veg being the largest on the platter. The US chose to separate fruit and vegetables but the UK kept them together; while the US lumps together all protein-based foods for just under a quarter of the plate, with the UK dividing them into milk and dairy, and meat, fish, eggs and beans. The US puts dairy to one side as a glass – presumably to represent milk, as drinking cheese might be quite hard. The UK puts a small space in for treats high in fat and sugar, but the US now leaves it out completely, unlike their previous pyramids.

- Cups – for portion sizes, many agencies have used cups. This works well for drinks but it is more challenging when talking about cups of broccoli, as people don't often measure this way. It can be done but many have different sized cups at home and get confused. A standard sized cup used to measure food should be 240 millilitres.
- Traffic lights – various versions of the traffic light system have been in use over recent years, some created by supermarkets or food companies specific to their own brand products. In June 2013, the UK government announced that it had reached an agreement with the major retailers to use one consistent traffic light label, identifying things such as total fat, saturated fat, salt and sugar and using a green, amber and red system to make it easier for people to make healthy choices (Gov.UK 2013).

RECORDING FOOD INTAKE

The UK government guidelines serve to inform people about the types and amounts of food they should be consuming, but what about measuring what actually makes it in to someone's insides? How can this be done?

FOOD DIARIES

Used to record everything consumed across a set amount of time, ranging between three and seven days, these are often used for health professionals to review someone's dietary intake and provide feedback with suggestions for changes. It is common for people to under-report or change what they usually eat when asked to do this, so as a method of analysing general diet it may not be completely accurate. This does not mean that they are not of use though, used regularly, over time they may serve to make people more conscious about the choices they are making.

FOOD FREQUENCY QUESTIONNAIRES

Again used to assess general food intake so that appropriate advice can be given, the food frequency questionnaire asks someone to select how often he or she consume from a list of foods. These can be useful but as they are based on memory they can be inaccurate.

HANDY TOOLS

Use the tools provided over the page to monitor food intake over time. Use both or just one depending on preference and reason for use. The first is a template for a food diary that can be used to record everything eaten and drunk on a daily basis. This has been adapted to be used over time instead of just for a few days as they normally are. As mentioned already, this may help to identify eating habits and trends, and also increase awareness of areas requiring change. If the client sends it to you to review regularly, it may increase motivation to eat well.

The second is a handy weekly shopping list and food consumption checker that can help identify strengths and areas for development based on the nutritional information presented in this chapter. Again, if used weekly, this can help to pick up trends and plan changes for the future.

FOOD DIARY

- Be as accurate as possible when recording what is consumed.
- Everything that is eaten or drunk (including alcohol) should be recorded. Note down the measures where relevant, e.g. teaspoon, one slice, one small bowl, etc.
- Remember the added extras like sugar in tea, sauces and second helpings.
- With homemade foods, write down the ingredients used; when eating out this will be harder but at least record what was ordered, rough sizes, etc.
- Start a new page for each day to help see trends on particular days of the week.
- Include details on times, mood and occasion such as 'visiting parents' or 'out with mates' to help identify key instances when problems may occur.
- Fill in the diary throughout the day rather than thinking back. This will make it less likely that things are forgotten.

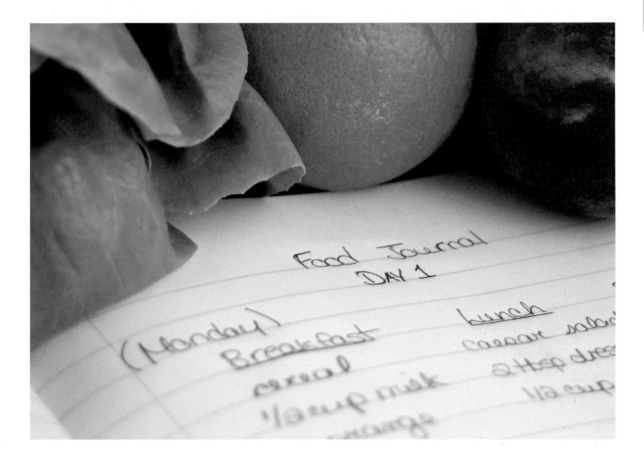

Day/Date:		
Time	**Food/drink consumed and quantity/ portion size**	**Notes – mood, energy level, occasion**
Breakfast		
Morning snacks		
Lunch		
Afternoon snacks		
Dinner		
After-dinner snacks		

WEEKLY SHOPPING LIST AND FOOD CONSUMPTION CHECKER

Does the weekly shop contain the following? Tick yes or no as appropriate.

Items	Yes	No
Does your shop contain enough fruit and vegetables to ensure at least five portions are consumed every day?		
Do you only consume enough food to make you pleasantly full?		
Do you tend to eat slowly, chewing your food properly?		
Do you have at least two portions of fish (one should be oily such as mackerel or sardines) and another source of Omega 3 such as nuts or avocado every week?		
Is the majority of the carbohydrate in your weekly shop from low GI or GL sources (see pages 88–90 for examples of these foods)?		
Do you get a good mix of quality protein sources, such as meats, whole milk and butter, eggs, nuts, seeds, beans, legumes, pulses and vegetables?		
Do you consume at least 1.5–2 litres of water per day? (Milk, squash, herbal tea and even tea and coffee count towards this.)		
Do you drink less than three high-sugar or sweetened drinks per week, including fruit juice, fizzy drinks and diet or lite options?		
Do you only eat processed foods, high in refined sugar and/or trans-fats as occasional treats?		
Do you have processes in place to control your eating when you know that you are likely to make poor choices, e.g. during times of altered mood or certain social occasions?		

'Yes' responses are good, each 'no' indicates an area to work on. Score your client one point for every yes answer they give. Total points out of ten. Once you've identified their first total score, work with them to identify ways to improve it by at least one next time or agree a target score to aim for.

POPULAR DIETS

Throughout this chapter the term 'diet' has been used to refer to a normal eating pattern, but it would be impossible to review nutrition without making mention of the numerous weight loss systems, or 'diets' available in books and online. While fitness professionals will not advise clients to follow any one in particular, it is worthwhile understanding what each entails in order to offer clients useful advice about the benefits and possible drawbacks of any approach. For a fuller understanding, it is always best to read the material on which the diet is based and then to review what the current research says.

Most people will attempt a diet at some point and this may be particularly true of people who join a gym or hire personal trainers as quite often they have weight loss goals. Many diets gain popularity because of their 'quick-fix' approach, but although they may help shed the pounds quickly, in the long run some may leave people heavier than when they started. This 'weight cycling', going up and down many times has been shown to be detrimental to health.

Many diets are actually based on some sound nutritional principles, but are then dressed up with a gimmick or marketed by celebrities to make them more appealing. It is this gimmick that will initially draw people in but ironically it's quite often the thing that will make them give up as they haven't got the time or willpower to be counting points, restricting certain foods or avoiding a particular food group. A review of popular diets or methods is presented below.

THE ATKINS DIET

A high-protein, low-carbohydrate diet, the principle is fairly simple; as carbohydrates are restricted the body is forced to start burning fat to provide energy.

Benefits:

- Reduced calorie intake.
- Decreased amounts of sugar, alcohol and processed foods consumed.

Drawbacks:

- High fat intake is still not recommended by government agencies.
- High-protein diet may cause kidney and bone issues.
- Decreased vitamin, mineral and antioxidant levels are possible in those that don't eat enough vegetables to replace lowered fruit consumption.
- A lack of fibre may cause issues with constipation.
- Ketosis can result in dizziness and bad breath.
- Challenging for vegetarians to follow.

THE ZONE DIET

This system is based on a specific ratio of macronutrients, 40 per cent carbohydrate, 30 per cent protein and 30 per cent fat.

Benefits:

- Encourages a reduction in junk food.
- Promotes intake of lean meats, fruit and vegetables.

Drawbacks:

- Difficult to maintain the correct ratio of nutrients in all meals and snacks as is suggested.
- The major focus of the diet is on macronutrient balance, possibly missing other important factors for long-term success.

INTERMITTENT FASTING

There are various takes on this method, involving periods of normal eating interspersed with very low calorie days. The 5:2 method is one such system, eat normally for five days a week and consume around a quarter of normal calories on the other two.

Benefits:

- Restriction of calories leads to weight loss.
- No foods are 'banned' with this approach.
- Short periods of time spent fasting may prevent metabolism from slowing as other low-calorie diets might.
- Normal eating days provide a 'break' from constant dieting for people.

Drawbacks:

- Severe restriction of calories takes a lot of willpower.
- People may be tempted to overeat on normal days due to excessive hunger.
- Focus needs to be paid to the quality of food consumed on normal days.

DETOX DIETS

Detox diets are alleged to work by removing toxins from the body, spending periods eating cleanly and abstaining from things such as wheat, dairy, sugar, meat and alcohol.

Benefits:

- They encourage consumption of a wide range of fruit, vegetables, nuts seeds and water.

Drawbacks:

- Detox diets tend to be short of many essential nutrients and may leave people feeling tired and unable to concentrate.
- Initial weight loss may be a result of a loss of water as glycogen stores are completely depleted; when normal eating patterns return, the weight often does too.
- There is little or no scientific evidence that periods of detox are required.

SLIMMING CLUBS

Each club has its own system; some involve assigning points to foods, being allowed a certain number of 'sins', or having 'free foods' that have no limitations.

Benefits:

- Today these are generally based on quite sound principles that encourage healthy eating habits and do not eliminate foods.
- Group meetings can help with adherence to a programme by providing support and encouragement.

Drawbacks:

- People may find points systems difficult to stick to in the long term.
- Some advocate the use of ready meals, shakes and bars, focusing on calories at the expense of quality nutrition.
- Some will find the weekly weigh-in a scary experience, and while it can motivate some, it does not show changes in body composition.
- Unlike diet books, there is a continuing cost for many of these programmes.

SOUTH BEACH DIET

One of a range of diets based on the glycaemic index, restricting foods that are high GI and replacing them with low GI alternatives. The diet initially starts by severely restricting carbohydrate intake before gradually reintroducing carbs with low GI options. In addition to this it recommends swapping saturated fats for unsaturated alternatives.

Benefits:

- Encourages healthy fats and a reduction in processed foods containing few nutrients.

Drawbacks:

- The severe restriction in the first phase can be difficult to stick to and leave people feeling tired and unable to concentrate, missing out on essential vitamins and minerals.
- Rapid weight loss often leads to weight cycling.

VERY LOW CALORIE DIETS

Known as VLCDs, these are diets of less than 800 kcals per day. They may be fad diets or used by medical practitioners in circumstances that require rapid weight loss, such as in preparation for surgery.

Benefits:

- If prepared by a medical practitioner, they should provide all of the essential nutrients.
- Lead to rapid weight loss.

Drawbacks:

- If followed without medical supervision, can lead to nutrient deficiencies and severe medical problems.
- Rapid weight loss may decrease metabolism and increase the likelihood of regaining weight.
- Increase the risk of gallstones as they prevent the gallbladder from emptying properly.

SUMMARY

You may wish to read this chapter a few times as there is quite a lot to take in and definitive answers are in short supply. Below are some of the key messages to take away for future use.

- Portion control is key. Regardless of the mixture of macronutrients consumed, the total amount counts.

- Eat low GI/low GL – controlling blood sugars and insulin levels, and improving sensitivity to insulin is essential in the long term for weight maintenance, health and energy levels.
- Omega 3 is key – oily fish, nuts, seeds and avocados help supply the body with this essential nutrient for health. It may suppress appetite and definitely has benefit for mood and the cardiovascular system.
- People are different – the controversy over the benefits of carbohydrates for some and not for others, why high-protein diets work well for one person and not the next, and why fat makes one person fat and one person thin may well be due to the fact that everyone is different. Certainly it has been suggested that some respond better to certain foods than others and that makes sense. What we don't know at present is how to definitively say from a science perspective what works best for whom. A bit of trial and error and learning from experience can come into play here.
- Good things come in little packages – those tiny micronutrients are key for health and make the body work better. Taken individually they may not improve weight loss, although chromium appears to offer help regulating blood sugars.
- Start the day right – eating breakfast works by controlling appetite and balancing energy levels, helping people make healthier choices later on.
- Mind over platter – getting to grips with the psychology of eating is vital to long-term success.

6

ACTIVITY AND EXERCISE

This chapter covers a broad range of topics related to exercise and weight loss. Firstly, it examines the evidence for the relationship between the two and then provides information on the importance of daily activities. Following this, various forms of structured exercise such as cardiovascular and resistance training are reviewed, and this is brought together with the latest exercise guidelines, advice on adaptations and a summary of the benefits, drawbacks and considerations of activity.

EXERCISE AND WEIGHT LOSS – THE EVIDENCE

Exercise is good for you, isn't it? Well, yes it is, it definitely improves health, decreases the risk of medical conditions and makes people feel better. Ever since the obesity crisis arose, exercise has been touted as the solution. This chapter looks at whether or not it has a part to play in beating the bulge and if certain types of exercise may be better than others.

Many have begun an exercise routine, bought a piece of home gym equipment or joined their local gym in an effort to lose weight, and the sad fact is that large numbers have not been, are not being and will not be successful. So is this because exercise doesn't help with weight loss? Not at all, there's plenty of research to show that exercise interventions can help people to decrease their fat stores. What follows is a brief review of the vast number of studies carried out; the intention here is merely to get a few key messages across.

EXERCISE VERSUS DIET

One study by Ross et al (2000) showed that people assigned to either cardiovascular exercise or dietary changes lost weight – both groups decreased stores of visceral fat and improved fitness. This provides some evidence that diet alone or exercise alone can result in weight loss. Interestingly, this study in obese men showed a greater weight loss with exercise than with diet, although this is not always the case.

In a review of nearly 500 studies, Miller, Koceja and Hamilton (1997) looked at the effects on weight loss of diet alone, exercise alone or a combination of the two. What they found was that, while there were differences in study design, all three methods brought about weight loss over a period of three to four months. A combination of exercise and diet appeared to be the most successful at keeping weight off.

Garrow and Summerbell (1995) also reviewed the literature, but they focused on the effects of exercise and dietary interventions on changes in body fat and lean mass in overweight men and women. What they found was that for people who went on a diet (a restriction of calories), for every 10 kg in weight they lost 2–3 kg in lean mass. If people did cardiovascular exercise alongside the diet, this loss was substantially reduced. This may account for the longer-term success of programmes involving both exercise and diet.

STRUCTURED EXERCISE VERSUS DAILY ACTIVITY

Do people have to go to the gym? Scientists have been studying this for a number of years, and the answer is no. They have seen weight loss and health changes in people doing structured exercise and daily activity outside of the gym.

One particularly interesting study looked at moderate intensity daily activities like walking and using the stairs for 30 minutes each day, compared to three times 30–45 minute cardiovascular exercise classes for women in their 40s with an average BMI of 33 (Andersen et al, 1999). At week 16 the groups had both lost around 8 kg on average and after one year both had regained only around 1–2 kg. Both had significant changes in cholesterol levels showing that movement is movement, regardless of where it is carried out.

A very well-known piece of research by Jakicic et al (1995), backed up by other research since, has shown that it does not matter if exercise is performed continuously or in shorter bouts across the day. This lends itself very nicely to lifestyle-based exercises, fitting short walks and movement in around family and work.

EXERCISE AND WEIGHT LOSS IN CHILDREN

While the focus of this book is on weight loss in adults, it is worth mentioning that research suggests that exercise has a similarly important role to play in fat reduction in children. Lifestyle activities may be just as effective as structured exercise (Epstein et al, 1985), and there has been a call for a bigger focus on 'play', especially for younger children, in order to make exercise more fun and at the same time help to manage weight (Burdette and Whitaker, 2005). Few adults would disagree that swinging on monkey bars is more fun that standing on a cross trainer for 20 minutes. This is not to say that more structured exercise doesn't have its place for weight loss in children; on the contrary, for those who may regard sports or group activities as unpleasant due to their previous experiences, individualised exercise plans can produce weight loss and improve health (Epstein et al, 1985). These programmes may also be helpful in improving self-esteem.

CARDIOVASCULAR VERSUS RESISTANCE TRAINING

This area has caused much debate in recent years, but the truth is there's probably room for both in an effective weight loss and weight management programme. It is evident that cardiovascular training leads to weight loss as you've already seen, but it can also decrease lean mass and, as a consequence, lower resting energy expenditure (Hunter et al, 2012). In the long term, this makes weight maintenance harder. Any weight loss lowers resting energy expenditure, as lighter people need to burn fewer calories to function, contrary to the popular belief that weight gain is due to 'slow metabolism'. Resistance training however, can conserve lean mass and as such helps to maintain slightly higher resting energy expenditure as weight decreases.

Cardiovascular training does, however, have health benefits in terms of lowering blood pressure, managing blood sugars and decreasing the risk of cardiovascular disease. It may surprise you to know that suitably intense resistance training can have all of the same effects, even in people in their 70s and beyond (Hagerman et al, 2000). If this is the case and resistance training can do what cardiovascular exercise can, but it doesn't quite work the other way round, then it has to be acknowledged that resistance is the more preferable of the two methods.

As fitness professionals, however, it is vital that you consider one key factor, adherence. If a client doesn't enjoy full-on resistance training sessions they will likely not stick to the programme. Training plans should be written based on a combination of safe, effective guidelines, personal preferences, wants and needs. Remember that the research shows that cardiovascular training brings about weight loss. OK it decreases lean mass slightly more but the client still loses weight, not to mention enjoying a whole host of other benefits. And if high intensity resistance training cannot be performed due to safety reasons or because of personal tastes, cardiovascular exercise can be combined with resistance training thus offsetting the likelihood of a reduction in lean mass.

SHORT-TERM WEIGHT LOSS AND LONG-TERM MAINTENANCE

It is generally accepted in scientific literature that people find it hard to keep weight off after losing it. Researchers now also believe that exercise appears to be one of, if not the major factor

in helping people to maintain weight loss. Active people appear far more likely to maintain changes than inactive folk (Baker and Brownell, 2000). This may be down to a combination of the physiological effects of exercise in terms of maintaining energy expenditure, combined with the psychological factors such as increased self-esteem and a more positive state of mind. From experience, those who exercise tend to feel good about themselves and less inclined to want to undo their good work with poor nutritional or lifestyle choices.

So now you know that exercise is important for weight loss, keeping it off, or for that matter preventing it going on in the first place, let's look at what you can do with your clients.

ACTIVITIES OF DAILY LIVING

Known as ADLs or activities of daily living, everyday activities that expend energy form a surprisingly important part of an effective weight loss and health programme. Fitness professionals should ensure that they spend as much, if not more, time focusing on a client's activity levels outside of the gym. The following statistics should help to explain why:

- There are 168 hours in a week.
- Of these approximately 49–56 are spent sleeping.
- Another 45 will be spent at work.
- Around 14 hours are spent eating.
- Those who go to the gym will average around three hours.

This leaves about 50 hours for life. Compare Peter and Jane's experiences on page 112 and you'll soon see how important those hours can be:

Peter

He crawls out of bed at 7:30, giving himself just enough time to get ready for work and jump into the car. He drives into the office and parks in the car park under work. His office is on the sixth floor so he takes the lift. Once he sits at his desk he stays there for most of the day, as he is very busy. His assistant gets him a sandwich at lunchtime so that he can eat it at his desk while he works. Occasionally, he has a meeting to go to or gets up to make a cup of coffee. When his day is done he drives home and because he is tired he puts his feet up and watches TV for a while. He spends some time with his young son playing on the Xbox before they have dinner, and then after his son has gone to bed, he watches a little more TV before retiring too. He sometimes reads in bed but is often so tired he just passes out straight away. At weekends he likes to go to the pub in the evening and watch the football on the TV during the day as reward for a hard week at work.

Jane

Jane always ensures she gets to bed by 10:30 so that she can get up early the next day. Twice a week she goes to a morning yoga class and her husband drops the children at school. On the other days she walks the kids to school and then catches the bus, where she gets off a few stops early. She walks in to work, climbs the stairs to the sixth floor and has some breakfast before starting her day. She works at her desk for a few hours before she has a break where she walks across the street to get herself a cup of tea. She always uses the stairs as she feels this helps to wake her up. At lunchtime she wanders across to the local park where if it's nice she sits on the grass, or if it's a standard day of English weather, she sits in the bandstand. In the afternoon she always spends time walking around the office talking to various people who have emailed questions to her that morning. When she gets home in the evening, she spends time with her family before dinner. In the summer they go to the park and play Frisbee or ball games, and in the winter they use their Wii to play tennis or golf. After dinner she relaxes by reading or doing a crossword before bed.

OK, so Peter and Jane are fictitious characters but hopefully you can see the point. Jane finds opportunities to include activity into her life as often as she can, ensuring that she can combine work and family time with movement. Peter has a similarly sedentary job but at present he does not find time to fit activity into his schedule. Jane's active lifestyle could contribute a significant amount to her ability to keep weight off, using a large amount of calories over time.

Twenty minutes washing the car could burn well over 100 calories, getting the recommended 30 minutes walking a day in could equate to 800–1,000 calories per week, and an hour's gardening could use up a staggering 400–500 calories, depending, of course, on how much the person weighs and the state of their garden. Even washing up and hoovering could amass a couple of hundred calories. As a well-known supermarket chain once claimed, every little helps, and if your client happened to do all of the above in one day, they'd burn around 1,700 calories – in theory at least, around half a pound in weight. It must be noted however that simply performing housework chores is unlikely to be vigorous enough to count towards the government's recommended 150 minutes of exercise per week. While it should

not be discouraged, larger muscle activities like walking and stair climbing should be emphasised to get slightly out of breath (BBC News, 2013).

Use the Daily Activity Changes table below with your clients to work out what alterations they could make. These are just ideas and clients should always be encouraged to suggest their own changes instead of us as fitness professionals telling them what to do.

Table 6.1	Daily Activity Changes
Current habit	**Change**
Drives/sits at a desk for work.	Take regular small breaks to get up and move around. Opt for a standing desk.
Drives into work and parks in the office car park.	Park ten minutes away and walk in. Commute by bike if possible, check out the Cycle to Work scheme or Sustrans.
Has a dishwasher or a cleaner.	Save pounds and the planet by washing up occasionally, get some exercise in by hoovering, or cleaning the windows.
Has gravelled over their entire garden or lives in a flat.	Get into gardening! Get an allotment, grow some fruit and vegetables and improve your diet at the same time.
Takes the car to the carwash, or just has a dirty car.	Get the bucket, sponge and wax out of the shed and get cleaning.
Drives the children to school every morning.	Look to make the school run an active family outing on bikes or by foot, even if it is only part of the way.
Uses every available mechanical device for transporting their body around.	Swap escalators, lifts, and travelators, for walking, pedal power, pogo sticks, space hoppers or roller blades.

Making a stand

It is not merely a lack of movement that appears to be bad for health and increases the risk of weight gain. Recent research has shown that sitting down itself may be particularly harmful, but that just standing up for a few hours more each day could have significant benefits.

Standing up may help to improve posture and alleviate muscle and joint pain, increase metabolic rate and contribute towards calorie burn, as well as decrease the long-term risk of heart disease. It appears that just standing may activate enzymes that trigger fat burning and people tend to move around more if performing tasks standing up (Macrae, 2008).

Work with your clients to find times across the day when they can get on their feet. The following are ideal opportunities:

- Standing desks – it is now possible to buy adjustable height desks for people to work while standing or seated. This way they can change the height throughout the day and spend a mixture of time standing and seated.
- Plan active breaks – it is important to get up out of the chair frequently. This can be done to make drinks, go and talk to colleagues or pop out to fetch lunch, for fresh air or for a small shopping trip for a few odds and ends.
- Have a ball – many find even sitting on a Swiss Ball a better alternative to a chair. It allows for more movement and for the core muscles to be activated. This can be done at work or while watching TV at home.

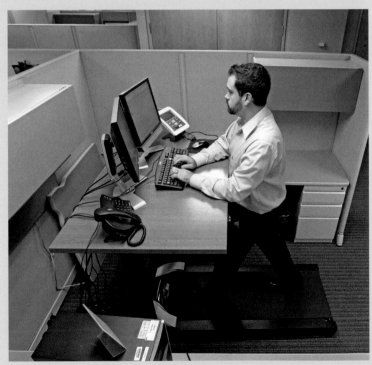

Figure 6.1 Making a stand: standing desks are becoming more commonplace, but some have taken it to the extreme!

DAILY ACTIVITY TRACKER

Use the simple weekly schedule on the following pages to identify with your clients the activities of daily living that they will perform as part of their exercise routine. You can record as much as you need on here, including time set aside for sleep, work, family life and other commitments, identifying how you can build activity into all of these (apart from sleep, of course).

An example of how Peter could change his daily activity has been provided for you. This has been kept as realistic as possible, with a little structured

exercise built into Peter's week as he is busy and has family commitments. Every day has a minimum of 40 minutes of activity built in by adapting his daily commute or by agreeing on more active family pastimes. His love of football is built into the routines, with him acting as referee at his son's training, playing five-a-side with work colleagues and using his exercise bike while watching the scores on a Saturday afternoon. Time is still put aside for Peter to relax and watch television or read throughout the week, and it is still possible for him to go to the pub.

Table 6.2	Peter's daily activity tracker						
	Monday	**Tuesday**	**Wednesday**	**Thursday**	**Friday**	**Saturday**	**Sunday**
00:00	Sleep					Sleep	Sleep/lie-in
01:00							
02:00							
03:00							
04:00							
05:00							
06:00							
07:00	Drive to outskirts of town						
08:00	Walk 20 minutes into work/buy breakfast and lunch for the day on the way					Walk to the local shop to buy breakfast for the family and a paper	

Table 6.2 Peter's daily activity tracker (cont.)

	Monday	Tuesday	Wednesday	Thursday	Friday	Saturday	Sunday
09:00	**Work** • Get up and move around every 90 minutes • Arrange some meetings in the local coffee shop to get outside occasionally • Have lunch outside in the summer when the weather is nice • Perform desk-based stretches once to twice per day					Breakfast	
10:00						Mow the lawn, wash the car, time to tinker with motorbike	Trip to the park with family/buy paper
11:00							
12:00							Read paper
13:00						Lunch	
14:00						Watch football on the TV. Use exercise bike for 30 minutes whilst doing this.	Shopping with family
15:00							
16:00							
17:00							Make Sunday dinner together
18:00	Take son to football training. Volunteer to be referee or linesman.	Walk 20 minutes back to car	Five-a-side football with work colleagues	Walk 20 minutes back to car	Walk 20 minutes back to car	Date night with wife – get babysitter and walk to local pub/restaurant	
19:00		Make dinner to allow wife to go to exercise class		Catch up on personal emails	Family games night, e.g. Wii or Twister and takeaway		Movie night
20:00	Dinner		Dinner	Dinner			
21:00	Watch TV						
22:00	Read before bed						
23:00	Sleep						

STRUCTURED EXERCISE

Now that you have an understanding of the importance of being active, it's time to look at the benefits of planned exercise sessions. There are various forms that structured exercise may take and each has differing effects. What these are and the part they might play in managing weight are covered in the following sections.

CARDIOVASCULAR TRAINING

Ever since Professor Cooper coined the term 'aerobics' in the 1960s (Cooper Institute, 2011), the idea that aerobic, or cardiovascular exercise is important has been ingrained into the psyche of society. Cardiovascular exercise can be defined as any exercise that involves the continuous use of the large muscles in the body. This brings a demand for energy from these muscles that can only be met if the heart pumps harder and faster and breathing rate increases. At a moderate intensity, carried out for more than a few minutes, the body's aerobic system does the majority of the work. To do this the body needs two things:

- Oxygen – delivered to the muscles via the lungs and blood vessels every time we breathe in.
- Energy – in aerobic exercise the body can use stores of carbohydrates and fats, and in times of need it can also break down muscle proteins, although this is generally not desired.

Cardiovascular exercise has always been thought to be essential for weight loss. The premise for this is simple; to lose weight people need to burn calories and cardiovascular exercise does this, therefore it must be good for weight loss. So, does it work? Well, like most things, you won't be able to find a definitive one-sentence answer to this. Let's look at what it's got going for it and some of the downsides too.

For

- It burns calories. There's no doubt about it, moving around uses energy and that can help with weight loss and maintenance. You won't see many overweight marathon runners so there must be something in it. Walking, running, cycling, rowing, skiing, cross-training and swimming all work many of the big muscles in the body and therefore use a lot of energy in the process.
- It keeps you healthy. There's plenty of research to show that cardiovascular exercise decreases the risk of heart disease, diabetes, some cancers and various other illnesses.
- It's enjoyable. Many people feel good after moving around, either because they feel pleased with themselves for doing it, or because they get a little boost of endorphins and hormones.

Against

- It may increase appetite. Research does show that if people perform hard cardiovascular exercise they may be tempted to consume more calories afterwards than they actually burned (Verger et al, 1992).
- It can be catabolic, that is to say, if too much is performed then it can lead to muscle breakdown, decreasing the body's lean mass and natural ability to burn calories. Find the right balance of training, however, and this risk is minimal, especially for those less fit just starting out. This is probably more of a concern for slightly fitter individuals who overtrain in an attempt to get fitter, such as members of

a running club, triathletes or ultra-endurance athletes.

- It can increase injury risk. Yes, repetitive actions can increase the stress placed on muscles, ligaments, bones, tendons and joints and as such increase the likelihood of injury. This is not a reason not to do it though, instead it is a reason to ensure that you get the programme right, progress it at the right level for the individual and vary it regularly ensuring that all components of fitness are covered.

The type of cardiovascular exercise should also be considered, as there are various methods to choose from, each having a different effect on the body. What differs is the duration and intensity of these sessions. There are various ways that the intensity of these sessions can be monitored. These include:

- Heart rate – there are a range of different formulas used for this, one of the most common being percentage of maximum heart rate (%MHR). A simple estimate of MHR is 220 minus your age.
- Rate of Perceived Exertion – this is a scale of perceived difficulty, with the client identifying how hard they feel they are working at any given time. The most commonly used form of this scale today ranges from 0–10, with 0–3 representing fairly light exercise, 4–6 being moderate to hard, and 7+ very hard. At around a four or a five a client should begin to get a bit of a sweat on and increase their breathing rate.
- Talk test – this simple test asks the client to talk while exercising. The fewer words they are able to say, the more intense the effort.

CONTINUOUS TRAINING

This can be broadly described as training performed at a continual speed/intensity. This may be fairly low intensity, as with steady state training, or higher intensity in the case of tempo/threshold training.

STEADY STATE TRAINING

This method has been of particular interest for weight loss over the years, as it corresponds to the legendary 'fat burning zone'. The fat burning zone is, to the surprise of many, an actual place and not a mythical land like Atlantis or Narnia. The fat burning zone is roughly equivalent to around 65–80 per cent maximum heart rate, a fairly light level for a trained individual (Anderson, 2013). At this intensity the body uses mostly fat to power its movement but that doesn't necessarily mean that this is the 'best' way to decrease fat stores. What this means is that the percentage of calories burned from fat is greater than those burned from carbohydrate, but because the overall intensity of the session is fairly low, the actual amount of fat burned in a session may be relatively small. Let's look at an example to show how this might work:

Bill does the following exercise session:

- 40 minutes cycling at 65 per cent MHR.
- He burns 250 calories.

As Bill was in the fat burning zone he would have burned around 50 per cent of his calories from fat, meaning around 125 calories.

Ted, however, does the following workout:

- 30 minutes hard interval training cycling at between 60 and 90 per cent MHR.
- He burns 450 calories.

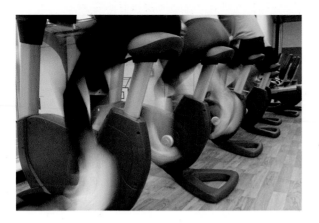

As Ted only spent some of the session in the fat burning zone, he may have burned around 33 per cent of his calories from fat, equalling around 150 calories.

The point being made here is that Ted did less work in the fat burning zone, burned more calories overall and even burned more calories from fat. Interval training clearly has a role to play then and will be discussed shortly, but let's stay with steady state training for a little longer. Clearly it isn't the most efficient way of burning calories but it does have the following advantages over intervals:

- Many clients are not conditioned enough to be able to cope with challenging interval training sessions in the early months of their exercise routines. Intense training may increase the risk of injury or, worse still for those with medical conditions, of heart attacks. Steady state sessions on the other hand are a great place to start with clients, gradually increasing duration as they get fitter and increasing their self-esteem as they reach new levels of fitness.
- Many are fearful of exercise and don't necessarily enjoy working hard. Intense sessions may

put them off and decrease their adherence to exercise in the long run. Steady state sessions allow the client to enjoy the experience as they should at no point feel too uncomfortable and should be able to hold a very brief conversation if working at the right level, allowing a good social experience as well.
- Lower intensity training may not bring with it the increased appetite that harder workouts might. In fact, steady state exercise has generally been shown to decrease appetite post-workout (Martins et al, 2008).

TEMPO/THRESHOLD TRAINING

This method involves continuous exercise at around the lactate threshold, the point between being aerobic (using oxygen for exercise) and anaerobic (working too hard to use oxygen for exercise), for a period of between 10 and 30 minutes. This is usually around 85 per cent of maximum heart rate for a fit individual but may be much lower for a deconditioned client. Not really suitable for those with low levels of fitness, this type of training is generally used for people trying to improve their times in events like ten-kilometre races or triathlons. For relatively fit individuals with no medical conditions, it certainly could be used as a good way to ramp up intensity and add extra calorie burn, but for those with lower levels of fitness the nature of the session makes it a relatively poor choice.

INTERVAL TRAINING

As you've already seen, this may well be a far more time-efficient way of burning calories for the right client. There are numerous different types of interval training though, so again the question has to be, are any better than the others? You should know the answer by now; it all depends on the person you're working with, their goals, their current fitness, their likes, dislikes, time available and, importantly, their current health. Let's have a look at various ways of mixing it up and see who they might be suitable for.

Interval method	Who's it for?
Long intervals, e.g. aerobic intervals	This can be used for everyone from the complete beginner to the advanced client. Longer intervals tend to be anywhere between three and eight minutes in duration and have fairly long recoveries between them, having a work-rest ratio of 1:1 for beginners. For unfit individuals they can be an ideal way to break up sessions when they are unable to perform cardiovascular work for long periods. For example, a less fit client may be asked to walk briskly at an intensity that makes them a little warm and slightly breathless, then to slow down to a more comfortable pace for the same length of time before repeating the effort.
Fartlek training	Meaning 'speed play' in Swedish, this method is literally random. It can contain any mix of intervals and rest periods desired and as such is a good option for everyone from the complete novice to the athlete. It can be used to great effect in weight loss sessions with less fit clients, asking them to work until they feel fatigued, letting them ease back until they have recovered and then repeating. Not setting fixed rest periods allows the client to judge the difficulty of the session and can be used to build self-esteem and ensure enjoyment in the early stages of the programme. The key goal at the outset of any good programme for an overweight client should not be weight loss or fitness; it should be to get them in the habit of coming back.
Lactate intervals	Not suitable for low levels of fitness, these fairly intense intervals ask clients to work at an RPE of around eight for between 30 and 90 seconds. The work-rest ratio for people new to this is 1:2, but fitter people will have shorter rest periods as they recover more quickly. The intense nature of these intervals makes them a good choice for calorie burning in fitter clients.
Maximal and supra-maximal intervals	In simple language, really hard intervals. Examples include: • Creatine Phosphate intervals – 10–20 second bursts with 30–60 second rests between each one. • Tabata intervals – 20 seconds maximum intensity with only 10 seconds recovery. This is generally repeated eight times before a longer rest period, and may be done in sets by those sadistic enough to do it again. These ultra-high intensity workouts have received attention in recent years, with science suggesting they may well be a great way to improve health and fitness.

BLASTING THE FAT OFF

The idea that very short, super-high intensity cardiovascular exercise may be good for weight loss and health may appear a little strange at first. But science shows that this may well be the case. Very hard exercise obviously uses a reasonable amount of calories in a short space of time, however, the work period is so short the actual amount burned during a session may not be substantial. What these sessions appear to do is fire the metabolism into overdrive, dramatically increasing what is known as EPOC after a session.

EPOC

EPOC is Excess Post-exercise Oxygen Consumption and refers to the amount of energy used in recovery and repair after exercise is finished. Steady state cardiovascular training does not produce a particularly large EPOC, but high intensity intervals do. They also improve sensitivity to insulin and improve glucose tolerance, decreasing risk of diabetes as a result, as well as improving the ability of the muscles to burn fat (Boutcher, 2011).

If you are working with an individual who has some experience of exercise and has no medical conditions or issues, it may be of great benefit to discuss high intensity training as an option with them. Remember to take into account something that the science does not, enjoyment. If they won't enjoy it they won't stick to it, and adherence is key to weight loss and weight maintenance.

RESISTANCE TRAINING

Resistance training is a term used to describe any form of exercise where the muscles of the body work against some form of challenge. In essence something stops them from moving easily, offering some resistance. The following are all examples of resistance training:

- Dumb-bells and barbells
- Bodyweight
- Suspension training
- Resistance bands
- Kettlebells

Resistance training should form an essential part of a weight loss programme for the majority of clients. The only exceptions may be very deconditioned individuals or those with medical conditions that make resistance training contra-indicated, for example those with both high blood pressure and diabetes.

Overweight and obese clients should consider including resistance training for all of the reasons above. Muscles use a lot of energy and it is no coincidence that body fat content starts to increase in people in their 30s and 40s as muscle mass starts to decrease. An increase in muscle mass can increase the amount of calories used at rest, and even the exercise session itself can bring about a fairly large calorie burn. Intense resistance training sessions have been shown to increase EPOC for well over a day following exercise (Schuenke and Mikat, 2002).

Injury risk, especially to weight-bearing joints including ankles, knees, hips and the spine, is increased with weight gain. Extra weight creates additional stress on these joints and, while weight loss is vital, strengthening the muscles, ligaments

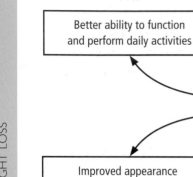

Increases calorie burning potential

Better ability to function and perform daily activities

Increases lean muscle mass

Improved appearance and self-confidence

Decreases risk of osteoporosis

Strengthens muscles, ligaments, joints – decreases injury risk

Figure 6.2 The importance of resistance training

and tendons around the joints can be of benefit in protecting them against possible damage.

While cardiovascular training raises self-esteem through increased fitness, resistance training can also help through improved ability in daily life, such as climbing stairs, getting out of a chair, carrying heavy bags and gardening. It can also create changes in shape and muscle tone, raising self-confidence further. This may not occur for those who are severely overweight due to the very high levels of fat covering the muscles.

Generally, compound (multi-joint), large muscle exercises that help the client to perform ADLs and give a bigger bang for their buck when compared to isolate (single joint) exercises, are preferred. They use more muscles and as such require greater energy expenditure. They are also generally the muscles used to in day-to-day life. Specific exercises to be selected are discussed later in the chapter.

CIRCUIT TRAINING AND OTHER METHODS

Circuit training is a method commonly used to achieve fat loss with clients. It involves the performance of a number of exercises in a sequence, usually a mixture of cardiovascular and resistance training, with a defined rest period between or, for the more advanced client, no rest at all.

Circuit workouts have a number of benefits:

- They can be adapted to suit any fitness level.
- They are time-efficient.
- They allow you to target all of the major muscles of the body in one exercise session.

- If they employ a number of compound exercises they can significantly raise metabolic rate and EPOC.
- They offer variety and enjoyment, and if done in a group setting, social interaction too.

Try the following workouts with your clients, or adapt them to suit their needs. See the specific guidelines later in the chapter about each exercise if you require more detail.

Beginner/low level of fitness	Intermediate/moderate fitness	Experienced/good fitness
1–2 circuits as able	1–2 circuits	2–3 circuits
6 exercises	10 exercises	8 exercises
10–12 repetitions per exercise	45 seconds per exercise	45–60 seconds per exercise
Minimal rest between exercises	15 seconds rest maximum	15 seconds rest maximum
1) Sit to stand	1) Bodyweight squat	1) Kettlebell front squat
2) Wall press-up	2) Standing cable chest press	2) Shuttle agility walk through cones
3) Chair dynaband back extension	3) Step-ups (low step)	3) Alternating arm cable shoulder press
4) Seated dynaband row	4) Standing cable row	4) Alternating arm row
5) Seated rotation	5) Wide-stance deadlift	5) Lateral step-up and over (low step)
6) Overhead press (adapt to upright row for those with hypertension)	6) Shuttle walks	6) Floor bridge
	7) Cable rotation	7) Box press-ups
	8) Bicep curls	8) Modified back extension
	9) March on the spot	
	10) Shoulder press (adapt to lateral raise for those with hypertension)	

As you can see, these three circuits encompass a broad spectrum of fitness levels, and that's because you'll work with a diverse range of overweight clients, everyone from obese clients with very low fitness and a range of medical conditions, through to overweight clients who are otherwise healthy and in some cases very fit. The first circuit comprises just resistance exercises to control the intensity and is known as a simple circuit. You may even perform a circuit with just three exercises; a sit to stand, push exercise and pull exercise for those deconditioned and new to exercise. The intermediate and experienced circuits include cardiovascular exercise and focus on large muscle exercises that help the clients to perform everyday tasks. Floor-based exercises have only been used for the fitter clients, as getting up from the floor will be challenging for some, and dizziness can occur due to postural hypotension. These can all be swapped for seated or standing alternatives if needed.

GROUP EXERCISE

Exercising as part of a group won't magic away any more fat, but it's worth considering as an option for clients who night benefit from the social aspect of exercise and from the support that comes with it. Walking clubs, specifically designed circuit classes, water-based and chair-based exercise sessions can all be used and adapted to suit the needs and fitness levels of participants. Should the group have medical conditions, care should be taken to ensure that they are safely monitored throughout the session.

OTHER FORMS OF EXERCISE

Because obesity can have a limiting effect on movement, flexibility, mobility and motor skills training should all form important parts of any exercise routine. These may have to be adapted as extremely overweight clients may find their range of movement limited by their size and shape. For these clients it will be important that mobility forms the mainstay of any early training as without this, cardiovascular and resistance training cannot be carried out effectively.

REST

As with any training programme, the right balance of exercise and rest is required. While the role of the instructor is to motivate clients to be more active, some who have not exercised before or for some time, may be keen to do more than they should as their self-esteem and mood improves dramatically. Instructors must explain the risks of overtraining and that rest is required for adaptations to occur.

PROGRAMMING FOR OVERWEIGHT AND OBESE CLIENTS
CONSIDERATIONS, BENEFITS AND RISKS

If you were asked to write down a list of all the benefits of exercise, you could probably fill a page with relative ease, and they are the same for overweight clients as for anyone else. Some, however, take on more importance for overweight and obese individuals. There are also generic risks to exercise, some specific to overweight clients.

A key consideration when programming, especially for those new to exercise, is confidence. It is common for exercise guidelines to talk of 'overload', 'exercise to exhaustion' or 'going to

Table 6.3	Benefits and risks of exercise for overweight clients
Benefits	**Risks**
• Decreases in fat mass. • Decreased abdominal and visceral fat, lowering risk of diabetes and heart disease. • Increased ability to perform ADLs. • Decreased blood pressure, cholesterol and blood glucose levels. • Management of or decreased risk of joint pain and damage. • Increased mobility and motor skills. • Psychological benefits including improved mood, confidence and self-esteem. • Stronger muscles, tendons, ligaments and bones.	• Joint pain or damage, especially the weight-bearing joints of the ankles, knees, hips, and spine. • Increased risk of coronary event or stroke. • Overheating and dehydration. • Decreased self-esteem and confidence with negative exercise experiences. • Diabetics may suffer issues with hypoglycemia, and damage to eyes, nerves and feet. • Fatigue

failure'. While these are absolutely essential to long-term success, the initial goal of any fitness professional should be to work with clients to make exercise a habit. Setting goals based on gym attendance or total minutes of exercise may be helpful in the early stages, as will focusing on exercises that clients find enjoyable. Exercise should be pitched at an achievable level so as to develop self-esteem, and the environment and time should be selected carefully to ensure comfort. Monday evenings in January at the gym may not be ideal for some.

OVERHEATING AND DEHYDRATION

Extremely overweight clients may find that they overheat more quickly due to the excess fat they carry acting as an insulator. Some will also find that they sweat heavily even at low intensities and can dehydrate quickly. To overcome this fitness professionals need to consider:

- Clothing – clients need to wear something that is loose-fitting and comfortable. The issue may be one of confidence at first, with some not keen to wear clothes that reveal their shape. Outlining appropriate clothing at the start and choosing quiet times or locations can help.
- Water – clients will need to ensure they take on adequate fluids both before and during the session.
- Temperature – ensure that the exercise environment is cool and where possible that the temperature can be adjusted to suit.

WEIGHT-BEARING

Excess weight puts strain on the joints and this is worsened during high impact or repetitive activity. Roughly three to five times body weight goes through the weight-bearing joints of the legs and spine during weight-bearing exercise. This means that being overweight by one stone could exert an extra three to five stone of pressure on the joints. It is estimated that one in five people have osteoarthritis in the USA, but that one in three obese people suffer from the disease (Kane, 2013).

Instructors can help by designing programmes that provide an appropriate mix of weight-bearing and non-weight-bearing activities. Clients should also be encouraged to ensure that they have adequate footwear for sessions, as cushioning may help to manage the stress on joints.

EXERCISE GUIDELINES

There are a range of bodies and agencies across the world that offer guidance on how much exercise should be carried out (Department of Health, 2011, Durstine et al, 2009, ACSM, 2009). The following section summarises guidance for the various components of fitness.

CARDIOVASCULAR EXERCISE AND DAILY ACTIVITY

How much should be done?	**UK Department of Health** 150 minutes of moderate intensity activity across the week in minimum bouts of 10 minutes OR 75 minutes of vigorous activity across the week. All adults should limit time spent sitting down. **American College of Sports Medicine** 150–250 minutes per week to prevent weight gain. 250+ minutes per week may be needed to prevent weight regain after loss. In general, adults should aim for 30–60 minutes per day, but these can be broken into 20–30 minute blocks.
How hard should it be?	**UK Department of Health** Moderate intensity – able to hold a conversation although increased breathing rate, temperature and heart rate should occur. Vigorous intensity – hard to hold a conversation, with significant changes in temperature, breathing and heart rate. **American College of Sports Medicine** Moderate intensity – approximately 60–75 per cent MHR for obese individuals, up to 85 per cent MHR* for otherwise healthy individuals.
What type of activity should be done?	**UK Department of Health** Moderate intensity – brisk walking or cycling. Dancing is recommended for older clients. Vigorous intensity – running or sports. Stair climbing is recommended for older clients. **American College of Sports Medicine** Activities involving the use of large muscle groups, e.g. walking, cycling, rowing or aqua aerobics.

* % MHR calculated by converting % VO_2 to % MHR using the Swain formula (Swain et al, 1994).

RESISTANCE TRAINING

How much should be done?	**UK Department of Health** Two or more days per week. **American College of Sports Medicine** None specified for obese clients but guidelines for the general population are 2–3 days per week, 8–10 exercises covering the total body.
How hard should it be?	**UK Department of Health** Strength training overcoming resistance. **American College of Sports Medicine** None specified for obese clients but guidelines for the general population are 1–2 sets of 8–10 repetitions to achieve overload.
What type of activity should be done?	**UK Department of Health** Body weight, weights training or lifting and carrying loads in everyday activity. For elderly clients, chair-based exercise and load-bearing activities such as dancing are recommended. **American College of Sports Medicine** Total body routine focusing on large muscle groups.

FLEXIBILITY AND MOTOR SKILLS

How much should be done?	**UK Department of Health** Two or more days per week. **American College of Sports Medicine** Flexibility 5–7 days per week, 10–15 seconds per stretch to maintain and 30 seconds to improve flexibility.
How hard should it be?	**UK Department of Health** Not specified. **American College of Sports Medicine** Not specified for obese clients but guidelines for the general population are to work at a point of mild discomfort for stretches.
What type of activity should be done?	**UK Department of Health** Tai chi or yoga for balance, coordination and flexibility. **American College of Sports Medicine** Developmental stretching to focus on increasing range of movement.

EXERCISE CHOICE AND ADAPTATIONS

The guidelines provide a useful framework within which to work. Now let's look at the specifics of exercise programming, namely what exercises to do, what not to do and how to adapt and amend them to suit overweight or obese clients.

For cardiovascular exercise consider the following:

- You may need to start with exercise durations well below the guidelines for deconditioned individuals.
- Consider balance when choosing exercises. Treadmill and high step-ups may not be appropriate choices for some if their mobility and coordination is an issue.
- Size and space – most modern day pieces of gym equipment are big and sturdy, designed

Table 6.4	Good cardiovascular exercise choices for overweight and obese clients	
Exercise	**Considerations for overweight clients**	**Considerations for obese clients**
Walking	Simple to carry out and suits short bouts of exercise built up over the day.	May need to be shorter duration due to limited mobility and lower fitness levels. In some very obese clients, it may cause chaffing so short bouts may be better. Shuttle walks between cones or lamp posts can be a good start point, and weaving in and out of cones can add an element of coordination and agility to mimic everyday life.
Water-based activities	Swimming or aqua aerobics use lots of muscles, decrease stress on joints and burn lots of calories. Some may feel uncomfortable in swimwear.	
Step-ups	Excellent for daily function and leg strengthening. Consider balance and range of movement and adjust step height accordingly. Lateral step-ups, sideways onto or across the step can be good progressions.	May need a lower step due to limited mobility. Consider placing them next to a rail/wall for support. Marching on the spot with knee lifts can be used as an alternative.
Activities of daily living	While these should be encouraged, fitter individuals will need more intense exercise to achieve overload.	May be a perfect place to start for less fit individuals and can be done accumulatively across the day.
Aerobics or circuit classes	Pitched at the correct level with the right exercise choice and adaptations, these can be extremely effective.	

to cope with the size of the population. Some older pieces of equipment, however, may not be suitable as they may be too small and some were not designed to take much more than around 20 stone in weight. Gym layouts may also be prohibitive for obese clients as equipment is often packed tightly together with small walkways. It can be embarrassing for clients to struggle to even reach the piece of equipment so think through location carefully.

- Comfort – the exercise bike is a great example of this. The saddles on studio cycling bikes and some upright cycles are not ideally suited to overweight clients. The recumbent bike may be a better choice in many cases because of its larger saddle and backrest offering support and helping to maintain posture.
- Impact – running, jumping, skipping and burpees are not ideal exercise choices for overweight clients. Regardless of what celebrity TV weight loss programmes do, high impact training puts a lot of stress through joints and excess weight exacerbates this. Impact is required to strengthen bones but those who are overweight will put suitable stresses on their bones and joints through exercises such as walking or step-ups.

Common resistance exercises may well be extremely useful with overweight clients, but there is a tendency to use overly complex or challenging exercises with deconditioned individuals. This may be an attempt to provide a wow factor, to work them hard to bring about weight loss, or because the fitness professional may see the exercise as too simple or not interesting enough.

For overweight clients with low levels of fitness and confidence you will have to provide suit-able alternatives or adaptations, so the following section has been designed to help you do this. You will certainly find far more complex exercises in other materials with much more depth of analysis about what they do and why. However, it is wise with many overweight, deconditioned clients to start with the regressed version of exercises and progress gradually to build confidence and self-esteem. Let's have a look at some very simple exercise adaptations broken down by functional movement pattern. It is assumed that you have some knowledge of exercise techniques so teaching points are kept to a minimum and start/finish pictures provided to guide you.

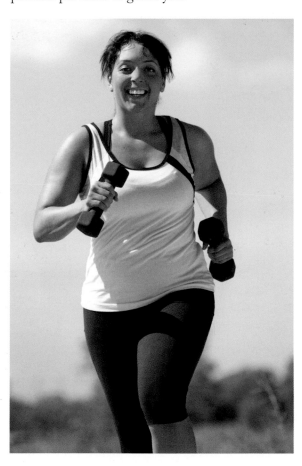

SQUAT MOVEMENTS (LEG AND LOWER BACK MUSCLES)
SIT TO STAND

A fantastic choice for clients, this exercise improves function in being able to stand up and sit down.

- Use a sturdy chair, place against a wall for support. Preferably it should have no armrests but for those who struggle to rise unaided, supports may be required.
- Feet should be flat on the floor, toes forwards or pointing slightly outwards.

- Clients should sit in the front third of the chair.
- Hands should be across the chest, unless needed for support.
- Maintain good posture throughout.
- Add repetitions, sets or resistance for progression.

PROGRESSION: BODY WEIGHT SQUATS
Considerations:

Can the client perform the squat with good posture/technique? If not, regress or adapt. A studio weights bar may be used for support or a wider stance can be used to ensure a suitable range of movement.

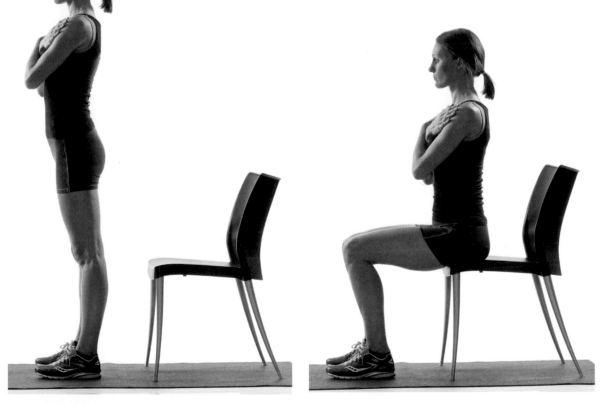

Figure 6.3 Sit to stand

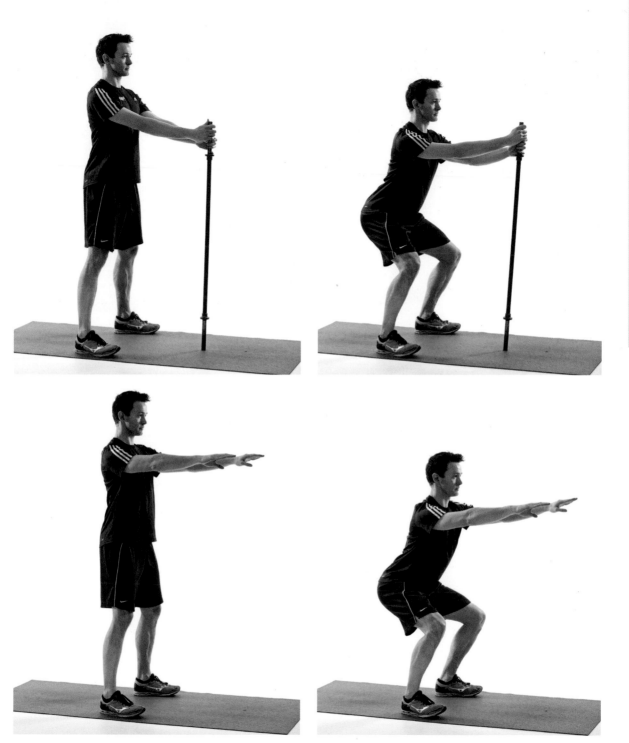

Figure 6.4 Body weight squats

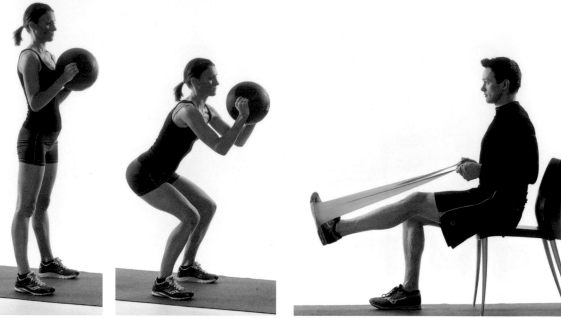

Figure 6.5 Front squats

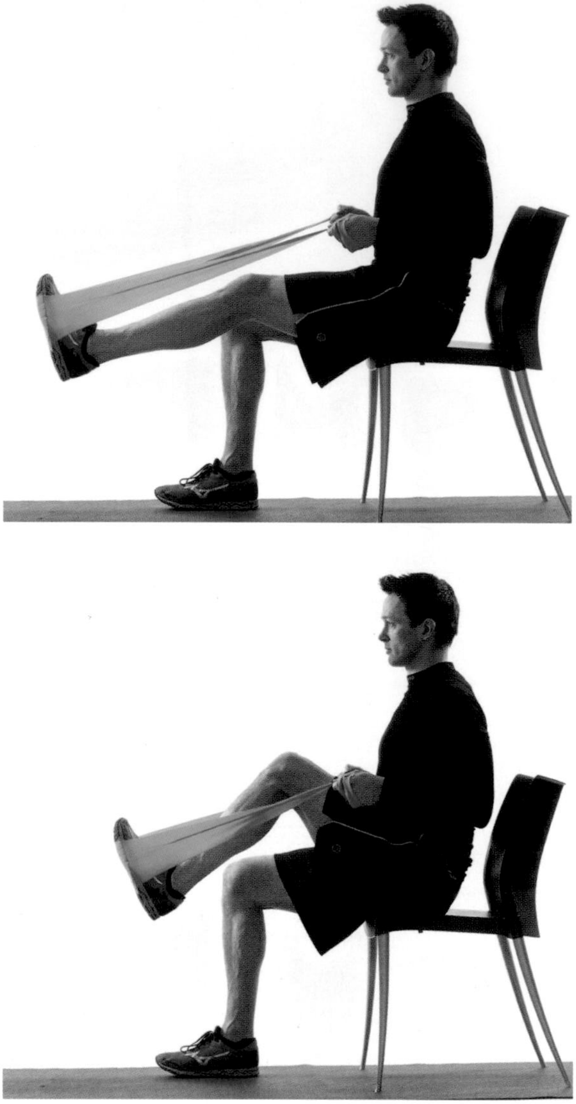

PROGRESSION: FRONT SQUATS
- Adding a weight makes exercise more challenging. Holding a bar behind the head often requires a lot of flexibility so a front squat may be a better alternative.
- Using a kettlebell, medicine ball, dumb-bell or plate can add some resistance while overcoming the issue of mobility.
- Hold the weight securely in two hands high on the chest. A wide stance squat can be used to ensure the body is kept upright throughout the movement, preventing the weight from moving forwards and increasing stress on the shoulder joints.

DYNABAND LEG PRESS
- Sit in a chair, legs bent at around 90 degrees.
- Wrap a band securely around the mid-part of the trainer, and secure it firmly in the hands.
- Pull the band taut by drawing the arms backwards.

Figure 6.6 Dynaband leg press

- The foot of the other leg should rest firmly on the floor.
- Bend the leg towards the body and then push through the foot to straighten, keeping the knee soft at the end of the movement.

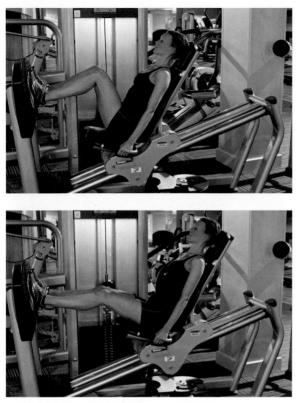

Figure 6.7 Leg press machine

PROGRESSION: LEG PRESS MACHINE
Considerations

Can the client perform the range of movement? Sometimes clients will feel 'squashed' in on these machines. If this is the case, decrease the range of movement or use an alternative.

PULL MOVEMENTS (BACK AND BICEPS MUSCLES)
SEATED DYNABAND ROW

- Ideal for deconditioned clients.
- Sit towards the front of a chair, legs bent at 90 degrees.

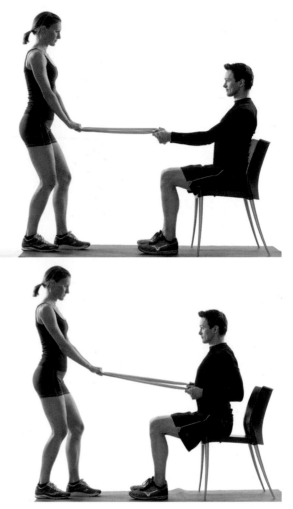

Figure 6.8 seated dynaband row

- Take hold of two ends of a dynaband, securing it safely around an anchor or having someone hold it.
- Keeping the shoulders relaxed pull the band backwards, keeping the elbows tight to the body to target the latissimus dorsi muscles. Using a wide pull will target the trapezius muscles.
- Keep wrists firm throughout and elbows soft when arms are extended.

133

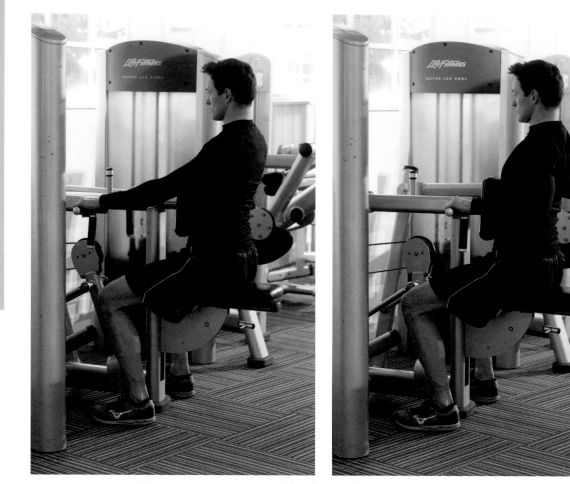

Figure 6.9 Seated row machine

PROGRESSION: SEATED ROW MACHINE

- The ability to adapt the position of this machine means it is often suitable for many overweight clients. Some may find the chest pad uncomfortable and so alternatives should be used.

- Narrow grip for latissimus dorsi or wide grip for trapezius muscles may be used dependent on the goal of the exercise.

PROGRESSION: CABLE ROW

- A great choice for overweight clients as cable machines can fit all sizes.
- The angle of pull can be changed to suit comfort, range of movement and goals.
- Keep wrists firm throughout and elbows soft when arms are extended.
- Ensure good posture is maintained throughout the movement.

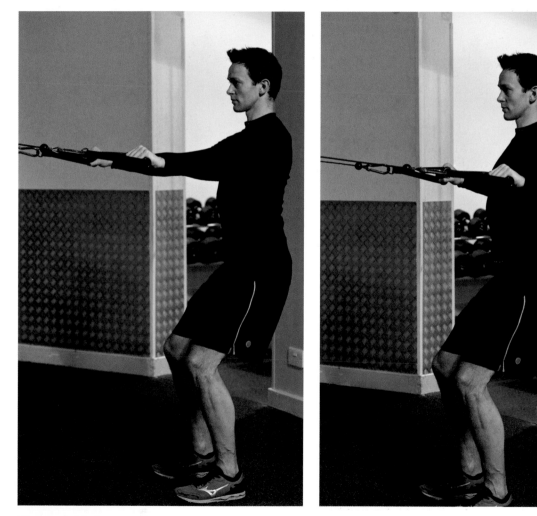

Figure 6.10 Cable row

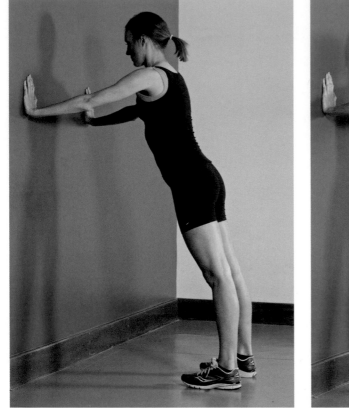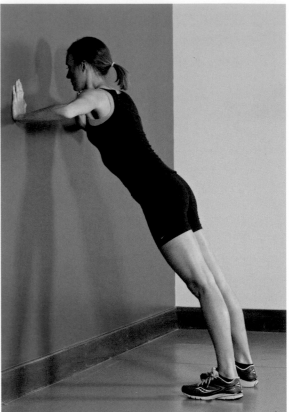

Figure 6.11 Wall press-ups

PUSH MOVEMENTS (CHEST, SHOULDER AND TRICEPS MUSCLES)
WALL PRESS-UP

- A great place to start to develop the muscles involved in pushing. Allows for a proportion of the bodyweight to be used as a resistance and reduces potential strain on the wrists.
- Place the hands at or slightly below chest height, one and a half times body width.
- Keeping the body in alignment, lower the chest between the arms and then return to the start position.

PROGRESSION: BOX PRESS-UP

- Increases the challenge by adding slightly more load through the arms.
- Be careful using this for those with knee and wrist problems or for people who find it difficult to get up from the floor.
- Ensure the chest lowers between the hands when performing the movement.
- Use mats for padding to ensure knees are comfortable.

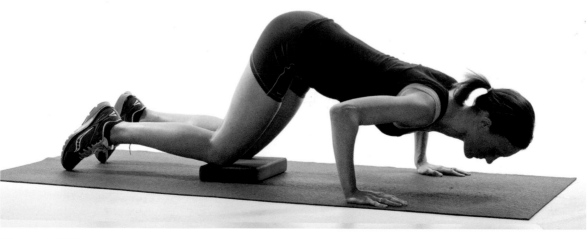

Figure 6.12 Box press-up

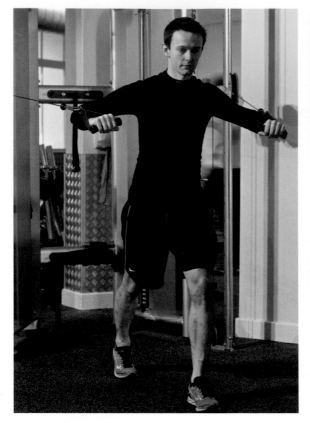 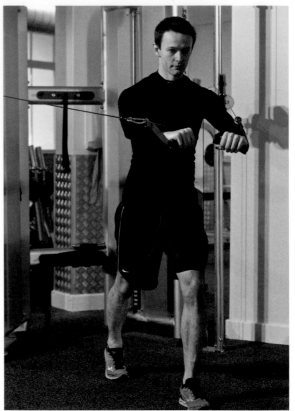

Figure 6.13 Cable chest press

PROGRESSION: CABLE CHEST PRESS

- As with row exercises, these work well as they can be adjusted to fit all shapes and sizes.
- Keep wrists firm throughout and elbows soft when arms are extended.
- Ensure good posture is maintained throughout the movement. Seated options can be used to help this and dynabands can mimic the same movement.

PROGRESSION: DUMB-BELL CHEST PRESS

- Dumb-bells can help to increase coordination and to challenge muscles further.
- Ensure that clients are comfortable on the bench used and can get up and down safely.
- Spot your clients as they perform the exercise for safety and support.
- Chest press machines can be used as an alternative but ensure that client can comfortably fit between the handles. Some are quite tight spaces and can be uncomfortable or embarrassing.

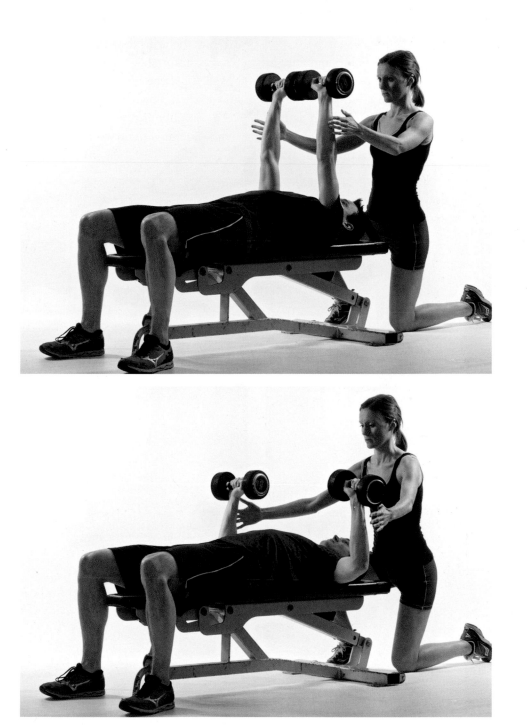

Figure 6.14 Dumb-bell chest press

WALL ANGELS

- Excellent for developing shoulder mobility in those who may have poor posture.
- Stand against a wall with good posture. Feet hip width apart, arms above the head as if at the top of a shoulder press movement. Elbows and wrists should be in contact with the wall.
- Draw the arms down towards the sides as far as is comfortable, maintaining contact with the wall. Once the comfortable range of movement is reached, slowly return to the start position.
- To simplify further perform shoulder press movements with no weights seated or standing.

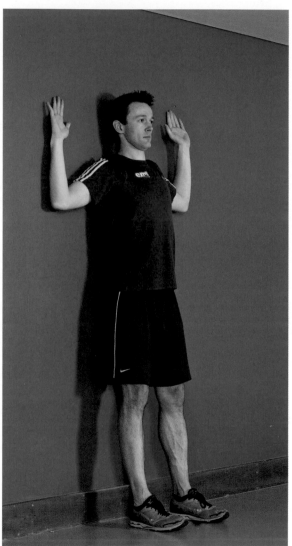

Figure 6.15 Wall angels

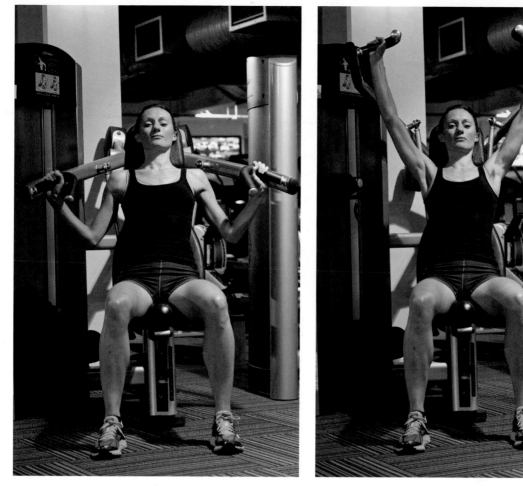

Figure 6.16 Shoulder press

PROGRESSION: SHOULDER PRESS

- This can be performed using a cable machine, or a resistance machine if preferred.
- Range of movement and angle of press should be adjusted to suit the client.
- The exercise can be seated or standing but the natural curve of the spine should be maintained throughout.

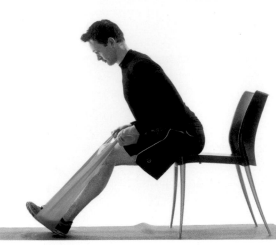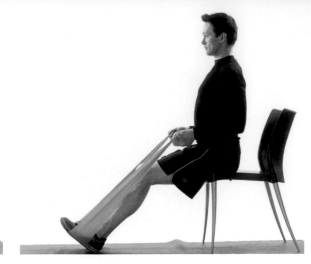
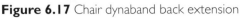

Figure 6.17 Chair dynaband back extension

LIFT/EXTEND MOVEMENTS (HAMSTRINGS, GLUTEAL MUSCLES AND BACK EXTENSORS)

CHAIR DYNABAND BACK EXTENSION

- Lying face down on the floor to do back extensions may be difficult for some. This dynaband alternative can help strengthen the erector spinae muscles without discomfort.
- Sit on the front third of a chair, feet hip width apart.
- Place the dynaband around the soles of the shoes ensuring it is secure.
- Take hold of both ends in the hands. Draw the arms back to add tension to the band.
- Hinge forwards as far as is comfortable with good posture and then extend the spine backwards using the erector spinae muscles. The arms should stay fixed throughout the movement.
- Finish in an upright position before repeating.

PROGRESSION: FLOOR BRIDGE

- Excellent for strengthening the hip extensors (hamstrings and gluteal muscles), if clients are comfortable getting down to the floor.

- Lie back, bending the knees to 90 degrees, feet flat on the floor, hip distance apart. Arms can rest on the floor by the sides.
- Push down through the feet, extending the hips upwards as far as is comfortable.
- If able to achieve full movement, stop at the point where spine and upper legs are in natural alignment, lower and repeat.

PROGRESSION: MODIFIED DEADLIFT

- Place a broom handle or an unloaded bar securely between two step boxes.
- Instruct the client to perform a normal deadlift technique; feet shoulder width apart or slightly wider, bending at the knees and hips to lower the body. The head should stay in line with the spine throughout.
- Choose a grip that feels comfortable and lift the broom handle maintaining good posture throughout.
- If preferred, shopping bags can be used instead, adding weight as required. This again ensures that the range of movement is less than a traditional deadlift but that it has carry-over to everyday life activities.

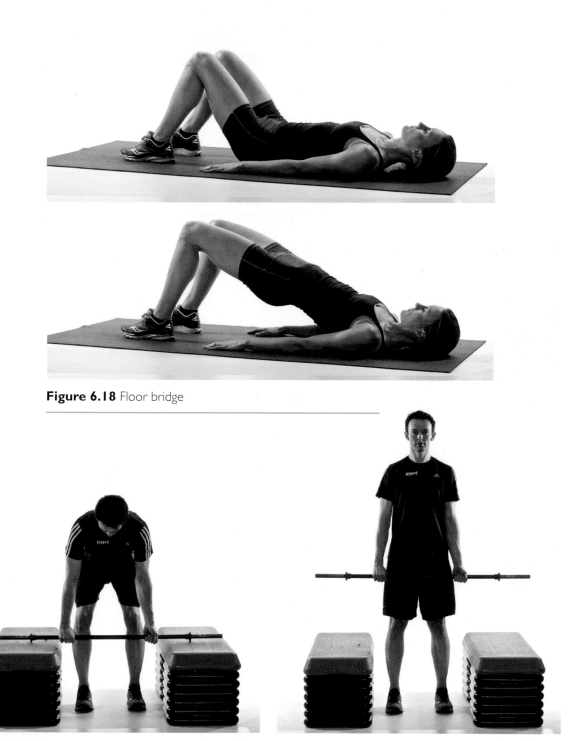

Figure 6.18 Floor bridge

Figure 6.19 Modified deadlift

143

PROGRESSION: BROOM HANDLE HIP HINGE

- Excellent for teaching clients about back care and lifting safely with limited mobility.
- Stand hip/shoulder width apart with a broom handle resting on the thighs as if at the top of a deadlift position.
- Hinge forwards from the hips keeping the spine in its natural alignment and ensuring the knees stay slightly bent.
- Stop at the point where posture would be compromised if further range of movement was used, and return to the start position.
- Head should stay in line with the spine throughout the movement.

PROGRESSION: WIDE STANCE DEADLIFT

- For many overweight clients, limited hip mobility can prevent them from performing lifting movements safely. For those that are able to, a wider stance may help overcome this.
- Stand with feet wide apart, toes turned out to about 45 degrees.
- A weight can be placed between the feet if needed – shopping bags, dumb-bells turned on end or kettlebells are decent examples.
- Perform a deadlift movement, ensuring the knees pass over the line of the toes and keeping good posture throughout.

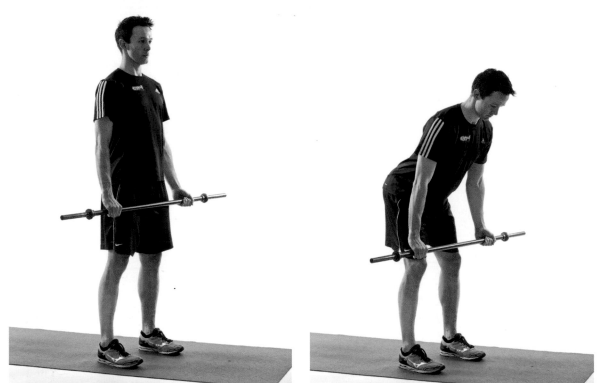

Figure 6.20 Broom handle hip hinge

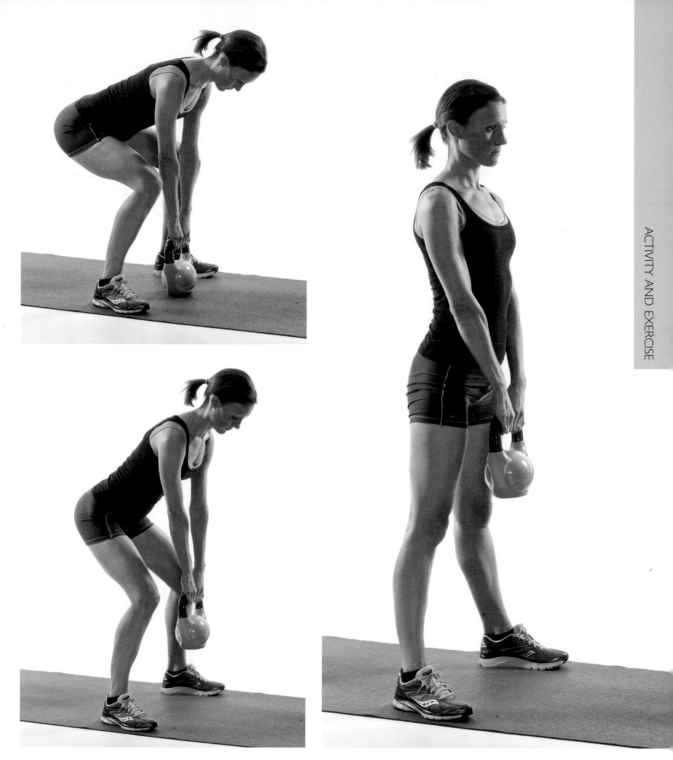

Figure 6.21 Wide stance deadlift

TWIST MOVEMENTS (TRUNK ROTATOR MUSCLES SUCH AS INTERNAL AND EXTERNAL OBLIQUES)
SEATED ROTATIONS

- The ability to rotate the spine is important for everyday activities. Many clients, especially those who have seated jobs or are largely sedentary, may have limited movement in their thoracic spine.
- Sit towards the front of a chair, legs bent at 90 degrees and feet flat on the floor. Sit upright looking forwards placing the hands across the shoulders.
- Rotate to one side as far as can be achieved comfortably without losing posture. Slowly move back to the start position and repeat to the other side.
- A very light medicine ball can be added as a simple progression.

PROGRESSION: CABLE ROTATIONS

- This is a good progression from the seated rotation. Cable machines or dynabands can be used to perform the movement.
- A range of grips and handles can be used but select the one that feels most comfortable for the client.
- For rotations to the right start by holding the cable out at shoulder height in front of the body, at a position of around 10 o'clock. Rotate through the torso, keeping the arms straight, to around 2 o'clock, return to the start, repeat for a set then swap sides.
- Progressions can be made by increasing the range of movement or adding the use of other muscles, such as the legs, to generate more power.

You will notice that the lunge pattern has not been included here. This is not to say that lunges cannot be performed with overweight clients.

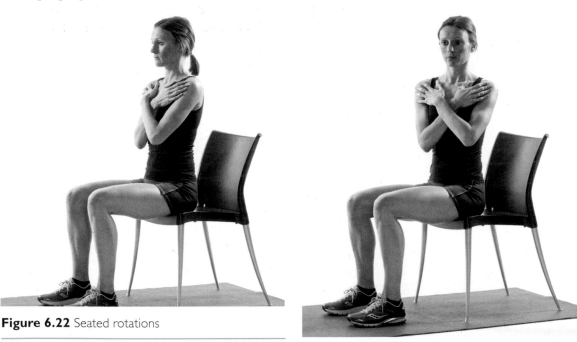

Figure 6.22 Seated rotations

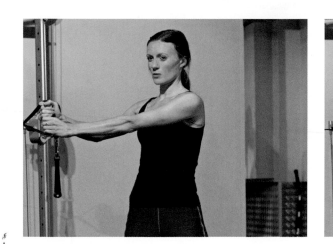

Figure 6.23 Cable rotations

It is merely to note that many will have poor balance and an excessive lumbar curve, known as hyperlordosis or anterior pelvic tilt. As such they may find lunges difficult to perform with tight hip-flexors. Hip mobility should be the focus until they can move efficiently, at which point lunges may become a suitable exercise choice for some. That said, flexibility and motor skill exercises can be adapted to suit overweight and obese clients.

FLEXIBILITY AND MOBILITY

This may well be the starting point for many exercise programmes for obese clients. A lack of movement makes challenging exercise almost impossible. Studies show that developmental stretching works, and that somewhere between one and four repetitions of a stretch held for 30 seconds can be effective (Pollock et al, 2011).

The following stretches may be particularly helpful in improving posture and movement for overweight clients. Many are simple but take into account limited mobility and client comfort.

STRETCHES
PECTORALS (CHEST)

- Step the opposing foot to the side being stretched forwards.
- Rest the arm on the wall at 90 degrees.
- Step into the stretch maintaining good posture. To increase gently rotate the head away from the stretch.

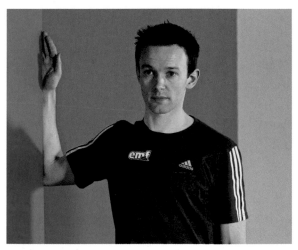

Figure 6.24 Pectoral stretch

147

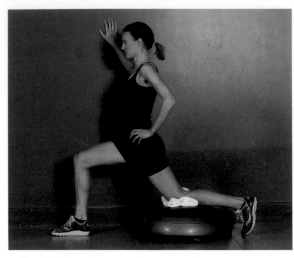

Figure 6.25 Hip flexor stretch

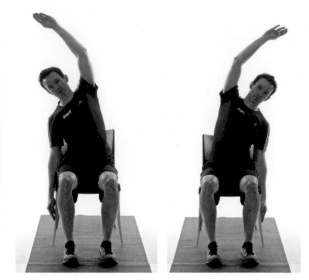

Figure 6.26 Latissimus dorsi stretch

HIP FLEXORS

- This may be particularly challenging due to increased tilt at the pelvis.
- Place a BOSU® against a wall and rest a folded towel on top. Have the client step one leg forwards, lowering the back knee onto the BOSU® while holding the wall for support.
- An upright posture should be maintained throughout.
- If the client feels comfortable they can increase the stretch by stepping the front leg forwards or tensing the gluteal muscles on the side being stretched.
- More towels can be added to decrease the range of movement of the stretch and make it easier.

LATISSIMUS DORSI

- Seated as shown, have the client raise one arm and gently lean across to one side until they feel the stretch.
- Repeat on the opposite side.

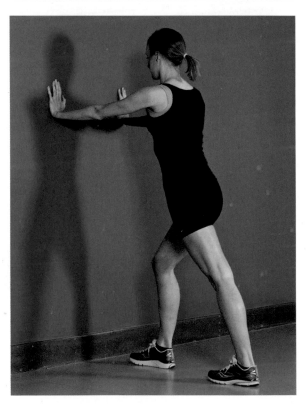

Figure 6.27 Calf stretch

CALVES

- Traditional standing calf stretches as shown work best for gastrocnemius.
- Flexing the back knee while holding onto the wall for support can stretch the soleus, or lifting the toes onto a low step while keeping the knee bent will also produce a stretch.

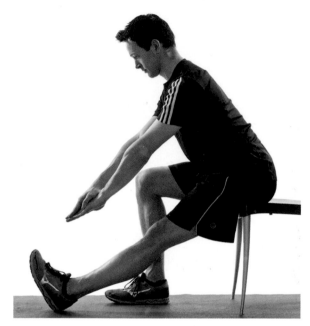

Figure 6.28 Hamstring stretch

HAMSTRINGS

- Seated stretches may be more comfortable for clients.
- Ask the client to sit towards the front of the chair and place one leg out straight, foot flat on the floor.
- Hinge forwards from the hips maintaining good posture until a stretch can be felt in the straight leg.
- Hands can be gently rested on the bent leg for support.

QUADRICEPS

- Rectus femoris, also being a hip flexor, can be very tight in overweight clients, especially those who are often sedentary. It is difficult to achieve a stretch from a seated position and the traditional standing stretch may bring with it balance issues.
- Have them lie on their side and support themselves as shown.
- Pull one leg back holding above or below the ankle as comfortable. It is likely they may not be able to reach and so a towel may be used or the trainer may assist if the client is happy with this.

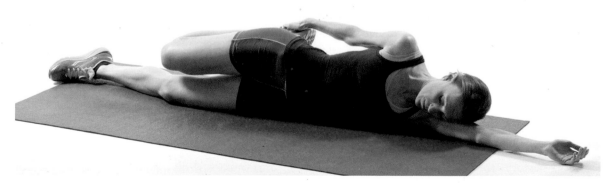

Figure 6.29 Quadricep stretch

TRUNK ROTATORS AND LOWER BACK

- Lower back muscles are difficult to stretch in many, especially overweight clients.
- Seated towards the front of a chair with good posture and feet flat on the floor ask your client to reach around to one side as far as comfortably possible. They can hold onto the chair to assist the stretch.
- Kneeling 'angry cat' back arches may be used to stretch the erector spinae if the client has no knee problems.

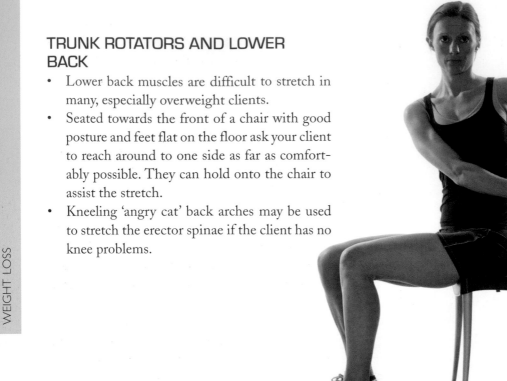

Figure 6.30 Trunk rotators and lower back stretch

Before an exercise session a mixture of standing static stretches, dynamic stretches and good old-fashioned joint mobility can be used to prepare the client for the workout. These should be chosen based on client needs and preference, considering balance, range of movement and intensity of the session ahead. Post-workout a total body stretch should be the focus, targeting tight muscles with one to four repetitions of developmental stretches. If as an instructor you feel it necessary to touch a client to perform these stretches, make sure you ask their permission first and discuss with them why this is necessary.

In terms of balance and coordination, the walking drills and resistance exercises already described will help to improve this. Coupled with these, you may wish to use one of the following:

Heel-to-toe walks

Although often used by the police to test if someone has had one too many on the way home from a night out, heel-to-toe walking can be surprisingly challenging when sober. Ask your clients to perform walking drills placing the heel of one foot directly in front of the toes of the other.

Short duration single-leg stands

As its name suggests, this drill involves standing on one leg for a small amount of time. A wall or rail may be used for support to regress the exercise. Good posture should be maintained throughout and if the client leans to one side or hops on the standing foot, the drill should be stopped to decrease injury risk or prevent the likelihood of falling. Initially aim for ten seconds on each leg and progress to 20–30 seconds over time.

LONG-TERM PROGRESSION

There are some key factors to consider when progressing exercise:

- Make incremental changes – do not progress any variable by more than 5–10 per cent at any one time. The body needs time to adapt, especially in those with less exercise experience. It is also essential that good technique and posture are maintained and that to build confidence, you choose options that, while challenging, your client will be able to complete.

- Change one or two things – linked to the above, this includes the exercise selection. Unless the client is not happy with their routine, there is no need to change programmes wholesale. Adapt exercises slowly over time and refrain from progressing onto complex exercises too soon. Remember, just because they are simple for you and you may not find them exciting, it doesn't mean your client feels the same.

- Get feedback – ask clients all the time about how they are finding the exercise sessions. What do they like? What don't they like? What would they like to do? What would they like to stop doing? How would they like

The Double Progressive Method

This is a simple tool to progress resistance training for deconditioned clients. It ensures gradual changes and allows them to build confidence over time. It involves the manipulation of resistance and repetitions to achieve progression. Let's have a look at an example:

Priya can currently perform eight repetitions on the seated row machine with 10 kg. The table below shows how you can progress her gradually over time.

Repetitions	8	9	10	11	12	8	9	10	11	12	8	9	10
Weight (kg)	10	10	10	10	10	11	11	11	11	11	12	12	12

As you can see, you keep the weight fixed as you add one repetition at a time across the sessions. Once Priya can reach the maximum number of repetitions desired, you increase the weight but drop the repetitions back to the lower part of the range again and repeat. You can do this a number of times to allow for gradual progression before changing the programme to avoid a plateau.

you to communicate with them? How do they want their programmes and progress recorded? Where would they like to exercise? When would they like to exercise?

EXERCISE FOR OVERWEIGHT CLIENTS WITH OTHER MEDICAL CONDITIONS

Many overweight clients will turn up having one or more other medical conditions. Should this be the case it is important to remember the following:

- Only accept these clients if you have suitable qualifications to deal with the illness in question.
- Ensure that the client has the all-clear from their GP or medical practitioner to begin exercise sessions.
- Use appropriate exercise guidelines for the conditions such as those developed by the ACSM (Durstine et al, 2009).
- Should a client have a range of conditions, be sure to use the lowest volume and intensity exercise guidelines for the conditions in question. This is vital to ensure that the risk of harm is not increased.
- Monitor clients regularly and send them back to their GP should any changes or complications occur, should they decide they are unhappy taking any prescribed medications, or feel that their treatment is not working.
- Work with the client to progress gradually and ensure they are comfortable at all stages. Ensure they are empowered to develop their own goals and exercise programmes with your help.

CASE STUDIES

Included here are two case studies of clients you may commonly see. These are designed to help you decide what exercises you may choose when working with similar clients.

BARRY

Barry is 45 years old and works as a taxi driver. He is self-employed so works long days and sometimes nights to give his family as good a life as he can. He used to prepare food to take with him for work but has got out of the habit of doing this in the last year or so. He also used to play golf at weekends and five-a-side football once or twice on weeknights.

Over the past 12 months, Barry has gained just over a stone in weight and says he often feels tired. He fuels himself on snacks and microwave foods from petrol stations during his shift and drinks Coke and coffee to keep him going. He says that once he has started his shift he tends not to get out of his cab much, except to go to the loo or top up with petrol.

He has a young son who loves football and on Saturdays they may go to watch the match together. He has never used a gym but has done circuit training with his football team in his younger days. His fitness test results were:

- BMI – 29
- Body fat percentage – 25 per cent
- Waist circumference – 96 cm
- Tight chest and hip flexor muscles

Barry's SMART goals are initially to lose half a stone in weight in ten weeks and to be able to play football for half an hour with his son without feeling exhausted. The following programme was agreed with Barry, ensuring he could fit it in with his work and family commitments.

Lifestyle activity	Initial goal	Progressions
Get out of the taxi and have a walk every now and then while on shift.	Twice each shift for ten minutes each time.	Three to four times each shift for ten minutes each time.
Play football with son at the weekend.	Initially aim for 15–20 minutes of activity.	30 minutes of activity.

Gym-based activity	Initial goal		Progressions
Warm-up	Five to eight minutes walking or X-trainer (as preferred) to an RPE of 4.		Possibly increase to target RPE faster, change equipment or increase intensity to RPE 5/6 as main session intensity increases
	Static stretches:	Chest	
		Hip flexors	
		Calves	
Main session	Circuit: • Eight minutes walking/X-trainer RPE 5. • Leg Press machine • Cable chest press • Seated row • Medicine ball rotation • 1 × 8–12 of each • Repeat × 2		Circuit: • Five minutes walking/X-trainer RPE 6. • Body weight squat (use broom handle to assist if required). • Cable chest press alternating arm. • Cable row • Cable rotation • Repeat whole circuit three times. Do cardiovascular exercise for a fourth time but not resistance.
Cool-down	Five minutes bike until breathing rate/heart rate returned to comfortable levels.		Five minutes bike/walk until breathing rate/heart rate returned to comfortable levels.

ANNE

Anne is 57 years old. She was always active at home until recently when she injured her knee gardening. She has had physiotherapy and has been given the all-clear but has lost her confidence in performing physical chores and no longer spends time in the garden. She has steadily gained weight and is now substantially heavier than she was. She has always found it challenging to control her weight but found that being active while eating well was the only thing that worked for her.

She has never been in a gym before. She once tried an aerobics class but found the movements confusing and was put off by the seemingly high level of fitness of the others in the class. She is able to walk to her local shops, which are about 15 minutes away but she is tired by the time she gets back so she prefers to take the car. She has contacted you to see if you can help her to lose at least a stone in weight and enable her to get back into her gardening, which she misses. Her husband has just retired and they are keen to be active and go on holidays where they would like to do a fair bit of walking. Her GP is keen for her to begin an exercise programme again before it affects her health.

Her fitness test results were:

BMI: 32
Body fat percentage: 33 per cent

Lifestyle activity	Initial goal	Progressions
Walk to shops	Initially do this daily but only 15 minutes to the shops. Her husband can pick her up so that she does not have to carry the bags home.	Aim to walk home once or twice per week with shopping.
Gardening	Start with light activities such as potting plants or hoeing weeds for 10–20 minutes 2–3 days per week.	Progress to longer spells of gardening or increase intensity of activities carried out.

Gym-based activity	Initial goal	Progressions
Warm-up	Use walk to shops as warm-up twice per week.	Increase to three times per week.
Main session	Chair-based exercise: • Dynaband leg press • Dynaband chest press • Dynaband back extension • Dynaband row • 1 × 8–12	Resistance exercises: • Sit to stand • Wall press-up • Modified deadlift (with shopping bags) • Dynaband row • 1–2 × 8–12
Cool-down	Chair-based stretches: • Chest • Upper back • Triceps • Hamstrings • Calves	Progress to some standing stretches if required.

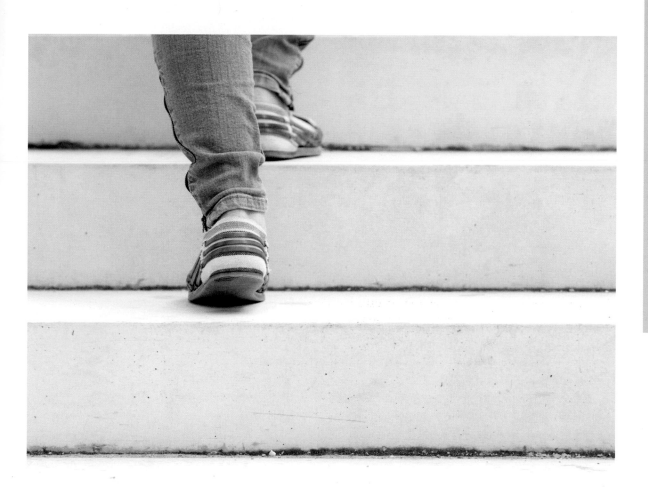

SUMMARY

- Exercise has a key role to play in weight loss and weight maintenance.
- Lifestyle activities like walking and climbing stairs, in ten-minute bouts across the day can be extremely beneficial. Housework is not intense enough on its own to produce weight loss but should still be encouraged and even standing instead of sitting can promote better health.
- Cardiovascular training works but where possible should be combined with resistance training to maximise maintenance of lean body mass.

- High intensity intervals are effective for weight loss. Consideration should be given to client preferences and health before opting for these.
- Resistance exercises should focus on large muscle, everyday movements.
- Appropriate exercises should be chosen for clients based on their experience, fitness, confidence and accompanying medical conditions. If suffering from the latter you should have suitable qualifications to work with them.
- Progress gradually and gather feedback regularly.

LIVING IT UP – HEALTHY LIFESTYLES

7

Daily activity has been covered in plenty of detail in the previous chapter, but there's far more to a healthy lifestyle than just walking the dog or taking the stairs. Lifestyle encompasses a wide range of things that can all impact on health and weight loss, often more than many would have thought. This includes alcohol intake, smoking (and giving up), sleep and stress.

The subsequent advice is meant to support those who would like to decrease or quit smoking/alcohol but do not need medical attention, or those who have mild issues with stress or sleep. People with more severe problems with any of these, or addiction problems should see a medical practitioner in the first instance.

CIGARETTES AND ALCOHOL

OK, so Oasis may have once said that these were all you need, but they were probably referring to their idea of a good night out as opposed to the perfect recipe for weight loss and healthy living. It is beyond the scope of this book to go into great detail on just how much these habits affect health, but it is certainly worth a quick recap of the medical conditions that use of alcohol and/ or cigarettes are linked with:

- Liver disease
- Coronary heart disease
- High blood pressure
- High cholesterol
- Lung cancer
- Emphysema
- Obesity
- Type 2 diabetes
- Bad teeth, nails, skin and hair
- Many other medical conditions

These negative effects will come as no surprise to most, yet recently it was reported that 44 per cent of men and 31 per cent of women in the UK consumed more than the recommended weekly intake of alcohol (Boniface and Shelton, 2013). That means on average nearly half of men are consuming more than one and a half pints a night, and a third of women are getting through more than two small glasses of wine each evening.

The recommended guidelines for alcohol consumption are shown in the diagram opposite.

Interestingly, in recent years there has been much support for the idea that drinking in moderation, within the guidelines presented above, may actually be beneficial for health, with a lower risk for heart disease than those who drink

Table 7.1	Recommended guidelines for alcohol consumption	
Gender	**Maximum weekly consumption**	

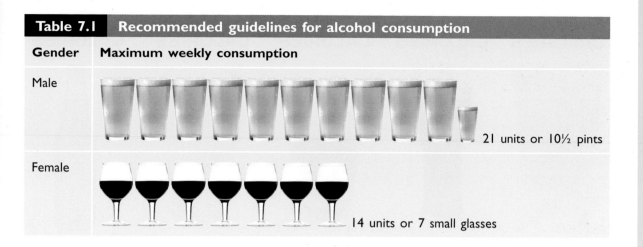

Male — 21 units or 10½ pints

Female — 14 units or 7 small glasses

nothing at all (Rimm et al, 1999). It appears that small amounts of alcohol increase levels of HDL cholesterol, known to be beneficial for health, and also decreases the risk of clotting. Like all things with nutrition there is a possible flip side, with a suggestion that even moderate alcohol consumption can increase the risk of a range of cancers (Bagnardi et al, 2001).

The benefits of alcohol may therefore be balanced with a fairly equal amount of risk. And there are other things that people can do to boost HDL cholesterol and decrease risk of clotting, like eating fruit and vegetables and doing more exercise. It also has to be remembered that, even if drinking alcohol is beneficial in small quantities, it is fairly heavy on the calories, and isn't directly used to make energy like macronutrients are. This coupled with the facts that it's certainly not filling and impairs judgement mean that it's easy to drink a large number of calories in one sitting, which isn't particularly helpful when trying to lose weight or keep it off.

How many calories are there in a common alcoholic beverage? This depends on the brand and the size of the glass, but here are some useful guidelines and a handy 'alculator' to work out how many calories are consumed each week from drink alone. Calories can vary with brand/type but those given below and over the page are based on averages taken from a range of common brands. For a more accurate record, check labelling information where possible.

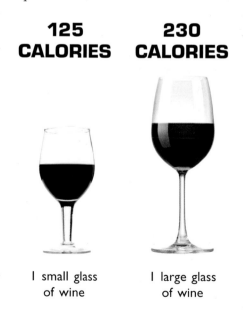

125 CALORIES   **230 CALORIES**

1 small glass of wine   1 large glass of wine

180 CALORIES	170 CALORIES	55 CALORIES	200 CALORIES	200 CALORIES
I pint of beer	I pint of Guiness	I single whisky/ vodka	I pint of cider	I bottle of alcopops

THE 'ALCULATOR'

Use the weekly tally chart to note what and how much is consumed each day of the week. Once you've tallied the amount of drinks for each category on a given day, multiply them by the calories listed in the table above, add them all up and put the total in the right-hand column. Being able to see this can help identify danger points across the week and also give an estimate of how many calories are being consumed. Use the results to agree changes for the future if necessary.

Alcohol isn't just a risk factor for weight gain and illness because of its calorie content. It has a number of other effects on the body that may contribute to the progression of disease:

FREE RADICAL PRODUCTION

Small amounts of alcohol can help to boost antioxidant levels. Red wine has received particular attention for this in recent years, with its high levels of resveratrol, a powerful antioxidant. Alcohol in excess of the recommended amounts however, will increase levels of free radicals, also known as reactive oxygen species and can increase the risk of illnesses such as fatty liver disease in the long term (Wu and Cederbaum, 2004).

HORMONES

Alcohol effects a range of hormones and the glands that produce them. It has been shown to impact blood sugar control (and therefore increase risk of type 2 diabetes), calcium metabolism (and therefore increase the risk of osteoporosis), and reproductive function (US Department of Health and Human Services, 1994).

SLEEP

Alcohol is known to affect sleep patterns and quality. You'll read more about sleep shortly but it's worth identifying the link here. It appears that alcohol can impact on the quality of a night's rest by decreasing Rapid Eye Movement (REM) sleep. It prevents people from entering deep sleep

The 'Alculator'								
Day of the week	**Pint of beer**	**Small glass of wine**	**Large glass of wine**	**Pint of ale**	**Pint of cider**	**Shot (single)**	**Bottle of alcopop**	**TOTAL CALORIES**
Monday								
Tuesday								
Wednesday								
Thursday								
Friday								
Saturday								
Sunday								
WEEKLY CALORIE TOTAL								

and as such is also associated with waking up more frequently (Park et al, 2006). 'So what?' I hear you say. Well, all of our lifestyle behaviours are closely linked and between them can impact weight and health. Poor sleep is linked to weight gain, and too much alcohol is associated with poor sleep – I'm sure you can make the connection.

If a client shows signs of alcohol addiction or if their drinking causes them health problems, instructors should refer them to their medical practitioner who can offer advice or pass them on to support groups.

Often considered alcohol's partner in crime, smoking is worthy of mention too. Hang on a minute you say, I know smoking is bad for health, but it's got nothing to do with weight gain has it? Well, you'd be sort of right. Smoking, or more specifically the nicotine found in cigarettes, is known to be an appetite suppressant. Until recently, scientists didn't know why, but in 2011 a group of researchers discovered the answer. They

The 'beer belly'

Everyone's heard of them, and they can be found in pubs up and down the country, but is there any truth to the term, or is it just a comical nickname? Well, you've already seen that there are plenty of calories in alcohol and it is thought that alcohol consumption increases appetite, but it's not clear that beer has any different properties to any of the other alcoholic beverages available at the bar.

Studies do show increases in waist circumference with alcohol consumption and that's no surprise. Some find that weight gain isn't specific to the abdomen and that increased fat mass will be seen all over, but one study did suggest that beer consumption might lead to more fat storage around the waist than if drinking wine (Duncan et al, 1995).

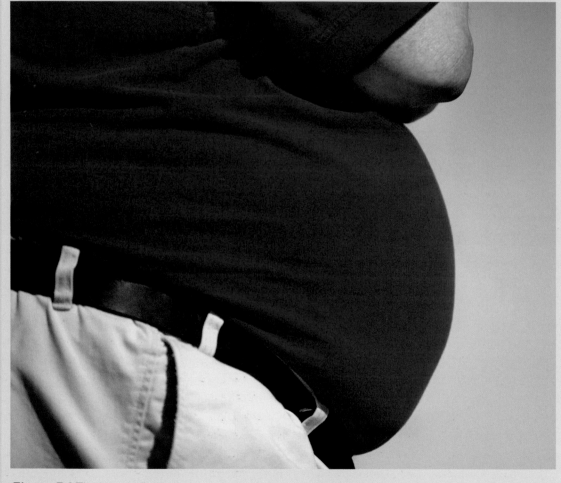

Figure 7.1 The beer belly

found that nicotine triggers a response from nerve cells within the brain, more specifically the hypothalamus (Mineur et al, 2011).

It's simple then, people should take up smoking and that'll help them lose weight? Or maybe the drawbacks of this plan somewhat outweigh the benefits, but there is a serious point to this. The use of nicotine patches for those quitting smoking may be helpful for maintaining a healthy weight. When someone stops smoking the appetite-suppressant effects are removed and that, combined with the fact that withdrawal can be a stressful time and they no longer have their coping mechanism to hand, can be a risky for weight gain.

There may be healthier ways to help prevent weight gain when quitting the little white sticks though. Chromium supplementation has received attention in recent times as it may help balance blood glucose levels and trigger appetite suppression in the brain (Parsons et al, 2009). See the chromium supplement guidance on page 96 for more information on how it regulates blood sugars and how much to take.

If appetite is increased when giving up, it makes sense that people should do all of the things they can to help regulate their food intake and increase feelings of fullness. This includes things like eating a low GI/GL diet and including protein with meals.

A scientific review looked at various methods employed to help prevent piling on the pounds when quitting. Weight management education and cognitive behavioural therapy were not successful and going on a very low-calorie diet worked only in the short term but led to long-term weight gain. Interestingly, exercise did not work in the short term but as a long-term method was successful (Farley et al, 2012).

Where the instructor recognises that the client needs more advice or support than they can give, they should refer them to appropriate practitioners or organisations such as the Department of Health's NHS Smokefree campaign (http://smokefree.nhs.uk/ways-to-quit/). This is a useful resource for anyone giving up.

The key messages to stay lean after giving up are:

- Nicotine patches may be beneficial, but do still contain nicotine so are not a long-term solution.
- Chromium supplements may help regulate appetite and blood sugars in the months after quitting.
- Eating low GI/GL and sufficient protein may help control appetite, and exercise should certainly be used to help maintain weight in the long term.

SLEEP IT OFF

It seems unlikely that lying down and closing your eyes could have any impact on weight loss, but the evidence is pretty unequivocal – not sleeping enough is a risk factor for weight gain. This happens because of a particular hormone called ghrelin. As you saw earlier in the book, this hormone is the one that drives hunger and it makes logical sense that, the more time spent awake, the more the body would call for energy from food to be able to keep going. The effect seems particularly strong in adolescents, who need more sleep than most due to the changes their bodies are going through (Patel and Hu, 2012).

Weight is also linked to sleep in another way, with obese people being at much greater risk of developing the condition sleep apnoea. People with this condition will stop breathing temporarily while asleep and this can happen many times a night in severe cases. Excess weight can cause changes in breathing mechanics and also effect the structure and function of the respiratory system. Sleep apnoea is not taken lightly as it can be deadly, and sufferers may be given breathing apparatus to use or might undergo weight loss surgery in an attempt to decrease the risk of adverse events caused by their health problems.

Of course, there are less serious effects of a lack of sleep too and they can play their part in weight gain. It sounds obvious, but less sleep will increase sleepiness during the day. Tiredness alone, or the subsequent changes in mood that come with it, can, as you know from Chapter 5, change eating behaviours. People who are tired are more likely to rely on high-energy snacks to get a boost, especially when they have higher levels of powerful hormones driving them to eat.

THE LAND OF NOD

It's clear then that people need their 40 winks, but what can they do to get them? This section is all about offering hints, tips and support for getting a better night's sleep.

NEEDS

Getting to bed early is important, but how much sleep is enough? This question has been debated many times by scientists over the years, and while the answer is not definitive, it seems safe to say that around seven to nine hours per night is considered ideal. Children and teenagers need a lot more and older people may require slightly less. Interestingly, while few would be surprised that not getting enough sleep can be detrimental to health, getting too much may also be harmful.

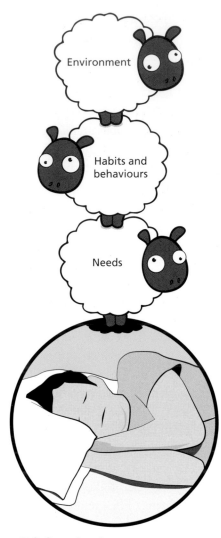

Figure 7.2 Counting sheep

The National Sleep Foundation (2013) points to research indicating that greater than nine hours sleep may be less healthy – seemingly too much or too little of almost anything can be bad for you.

The actual amount of sleep needed for each person will vary, and be influenced by a number of important factors including:

- Sleep debt – this is a term used to describe the accumulation of missed sleep over time. The exact meaning of the term and how this can be overcome are the source of debate, but it seems clear that without enough sleep people experience physical and psychological symptoms. It seems that sleep debt can be made up over time by returning to good sleep habits (Van Dongen et al, 2003).
- Exercise – those who have exercised hard during the day may need more sleep to recover from their efforts.
- Stress – mental stress, much like physical challenges, exerts the body. Ever noticed how tiring a mentally stressful day can be? In fact, many people exercise to feel less tired.
- Time of year – nearer the poles the dramatic changes in the length of days from season to season can play a big role in energy levels. It is common to need more sleep in those dark winter months.
- Illness – colds, flus, viruses and the like can sap energy levels and increase the need for sleep and recovery.

HABITS AND BEHAVIOURS

Getting into good habits is a very helpful way to ensure enough sleep. Suggest the following to clients to set effective daily routines:

- Set a bedtime and stick to it. Aim to be asleep by 11 pm, which means being in bed by around 10:30 pm.
- Wind down before bed. Switch off the computer and TV, stop working and take time to relax by reading, listening to music or having a bath.
- Avoid stimulants like tea and coffee later in the day.

- Drink in moderation – you've already seen how sleep quality is effected by alcohol.

ENVIRONMENT

The right surroundings can make a big difference.

- Go dark – light stimulates the body, increasing wakefulness. Even a tiny speck of light on the skin has been shown to increase levels of fight or flight hormones so it's important to switch off all light sources, including standby lights and chargers where possible. If able, use curtains that block out light sources.
- Chill – not just the relaxing type, but temperature too. A cooler environment is better for a restful night.
- Make the bedroom a peaceful place. A little bit of Feng Shui can help, as if the bedroom is the place of work as well as sleep, it's easy to associate it with stress and make it hard to switch off.

If all of this fails to work, then there's always the age-old method of counting sheep. It is said to originate from the fact that shepherds had to count their flock before bedtime, and rumour had it that it was such a boring task that it used to help them nod off. Disappointingly though, the only bit of research I found that tests this notion suggests it doesn't work. When groups were either asked to do nothing, imagine themselves on a tropical beach or count sheep, numbering the flock came off worst in terms of how long it took to get to sleep. The study's authors proposed that this may have been due to the fact that it was so dull that an individual could not do it for long enough to help them drift off, but the thought of laying on golden sands with the waves gently lapping at their feet may just do the trick (Harvey and Payne, 2002).

STRESS

The very mention of the word stress brings to mind a frazzled individual, sat at their desk pulling their hair out as the work piles up, or a parent juggling family life with work, shopping, cooking tea and trying desperately to fit in some time for themselves.

But what does stress actually mean? The *Oxford Dictionary* (2013) defines it as 'something that causes strain or tension.' Interestingly though, it also gives the definition that would spring to mind for most these days; 'a state of mental or emotional strain or tension resulting from adverse or demanding circumstances'. And it is this definition that will form the basis of the advice to follow.

The Health and Safety Executive (2012) said that there were 428,000 cases of work-related stress in 2011/2012, and that the most common occupations to suffer were health professionals and those in education. Shhhh! Don't tell all those fitness instructors and personal trainers.

Like many of the topics in this book, there are volumes worth of information to be read and written on the subject of stress. The focus of the next few pages, however, is on the relationship between stress and weight gain. This is more

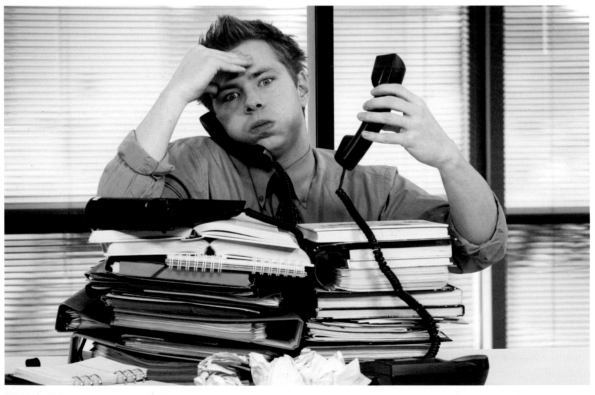

Figure 7.3 Life stress

complex than you may imagine, as stress can impact on both psychological and physiological factors. It is known to have an effect on:

- Appetite.
- Energy levels, mood and subsequent eating behaviour.
- Hormone levels, including cortisol and insulin.
- Other unhealthy behaviours, including being sedentary, drinking alcohol and drug-taking.

APPETITE

Ask most people and they will tell you that their appetite changes when they feel stressed. Some will tell you that they feel hungry less often, eat less and are prone to losing weight in times of stress. Others will say the exact opposite; tending to gravitate towards chocolate and ice cream when times get tough. Although 'comfort eating' is generally thought of as a female trait, researchers have observed it in both men and women (Kandiah et al, 2005; Oliver and Wardle, 1999).

ENERGY LEVELS, MOOD AND SUBSEQUENT EATING BEHAVIOUR

Stress is … well, it's stressful, and it's tiring. People will often talk of being 'drained', 'shattered' or 'exhausted' after a stressful day or time. You've seen already in Chapter 5 how mood can effect eating behaviour, and one of the obvious consequences can be a desire for high-energy foods. High-sugar, high-GI foods cause insulin spikes and subsequent crashes, exasperating tiredness, which in turn effects mood further and can become a vicious circle. If the behaviour continues, increased stores of fat are likely.

THE NEGATIVE CYCLE OF STRESS

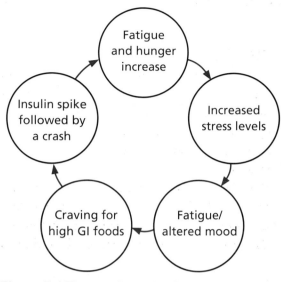

Figure 7.4 The negative cycle of stress

HORMONE LEVELS

Intrinsically linked to all of this are changes in important hormones regulating mood, appetite and energy storage. Changes in cortisol and insulin levels due to psychological stress are common and this brings about increased hunger and a strong likelihood that more calories will be taken on board. When exposed to a stressful situation in laboratory tests, those whose cortisol levels rose more dramatically, consistently ate more calories afterwards (Epel et al, 2001). These hormone changes lead to a cascade of events that increase the likelihood of fat storage and the risk of type 2 diabetes (Epel, 2009). In turn, diabetes causes a host of physiological problems including damage to nerves, muscles and organs, as well as changes in cholesterol and blood pressure levels. Because of the metabolic changes, people may find it increasingly difficult to lose weight.

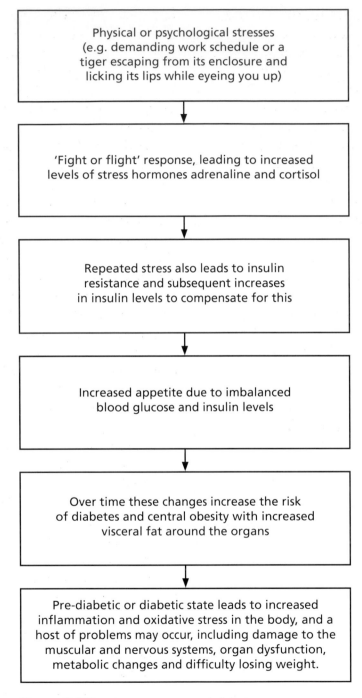

Figure 7.5 The stress response and diabetes

OTHER UNHEALTHY BEHAVIOURS

It's not just eating patterns that can change in times of stress. Every individual may have a different response and in many cases the choice of coping mechanism may not be a healthy one. Some may lose the motivation to exercise, or even to move, some may turn to alcohol to relax or distract them from their worries and, worse still, some may opt for drugs in extreme cases. Obviously, it is beyond the professional area of expertise of the fitness professional to offer support in severe cases, and referral to a medical practitioner is essential.

If mild stress is causing someone to be inactive then the creation of an appropriate exercise programme can be a great help for both stress relief and managing the risks of weight gain.

THE POSITIVE CYCLE OF STRESS MANAGEMENT

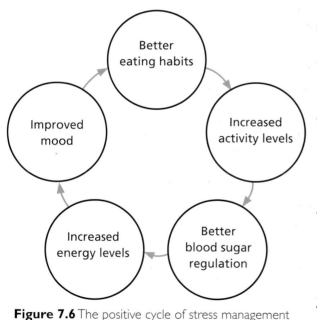

Figure 7.6 The positive cycle of stress management

STRESS MANAGEMENT

As the stress response is different for everyone, so must the methods be that they use to manage it. As fitness professionals, it is important to assess whether or not you are able to work with the client to support them in developing stress management programmes. Those with more severe stress that is affecting their psychological state or having adverse effects on their physiology that may pose a risk to them should be referred to a medical practitioner. It will then be up to the GP to decide the best course of treatment. This may be medication, therapy or entry into an exercise referral scheme. If the latter is the case, fitness professionals with appropriate qualifications can work with the client to agree an exercise and lifestyle programme based on suitable guidelines. For clients for whom GPs simply recommend changes in lifestyle, personal trainers can work with them as they would other clients, adapting advice to suit their needs.

For those referred by their GP, the ACSM (2009) recommend the following for exercise regimes:

- Consider the effects of the medications the client is taking and adapt the session accordingly.
- Assess the client's physical and functional ability before beginning an exercise programme, including tests for cardiovascular fitness, strength, flexibility and neuromuscular function such as balance and coordination.
- Use the exercise guidelines for cardiovascular and resistance exercise for healthy populations as goals to work towards, adjusting the rate of progression based on any condition-specific considerations.
- As clients may be unfamiliar with resistance training, the early focus should be on cardio-

vascular exercise, which has a good evidence base for use. Introduce resistance training slowly, progressing an exercise when the client is able to complete two repetitions more than originally planned.

- Monitor clients closely, especially in the early stage of a programme. They may have been sedentary for some time and therefore at an increased risk of injury or of giving up should they find the exercise programmes too challenging.

For those with lower levels of stress not referred by their GP, exercise is still extremely beneficial.

There are very few hard and fast guidelines about exactly what sort of exercise should be done, but the following should serve to help when creating programmes.

CARDIOVASCULAR EXERCISE

People with mild stress, anxiety and depression can become sedentary (Paluska and Schwenk, 2000). Exercise is therefore important not just to help with managing the condition, but because it will decrease the risk of weight gain and the development of other medical conditions in the long term. People often report mood-altering effects of cardiovascular exercise and while the

---

Stress and the brain

Ever wondered what goes on in the grey matter that causes someone to change behaviour so radically during times of stress? It appears that the brain's wiring may be a little faulty when under pressure, causing patterns of behaviour that may not normally be expected or seen.

Changes in the activation of an area of the brain known as the putamen, may decrease reward signalling and this could mean that people opt for foods or behaviours that seek to satisfy them more than usual, with tastier foods and high carbohydrate content preferred (Born et al, 2010).

The amygdala in the brain also plays a major role. It helps people to make snap decisions in instances that might be stressful or dangerous, in an effort to preserve life. Without it, the brain would have to process the situation, and those valuable few seconds might mean the difference between life and death. Imagine you step out into the road, see something hurtling towards you out of the corner of your eye, and instantly throw yourself backwards like an Olympic gymnast, tumbling into a heap on the floor. If it had been a car, your amygdala's ability to help you react quickly may have just saved your life. As it turned out, it was a Labrador chasing a tennis ball thrown by its owner. But if you'd had to look, process the information, and it had turned out it to be a businessman in his Audi, speeding to a meeting he was late for, then you'd have had more than sore knees and bruised pride.

Quick decisions without thought are great in times of danger, but irrational actions not thought through after other stressors may not be. Poor food choices that satisfy the pleasure-sensing areas of the brain may seem like a great idea at the time, but when rational thought kicks in shortly after, people often feel guilty about their actions, leading them to feel down and making it worse as the negative cycle of stress goes round again.

exact mechanisms for this are not fully understood yet, there may be a range of possible causes:

- Changes in levels of chemicals – exercise can affect the levels of hormones in the bloodstream, such as adrenaline, as well as increasing neurotransmitters in the brain such as dopamine and, of course, endorphins. These have painkiller-like effects, bringing about a state of relaxation.
- Distraction – many will say that exercise helps to take their mind off their daily stresses. Some will call it 'me time', enabling them to show themselves a bit of TLC. Others may say that rather than distracting them, time away from a problem helps them to think it through more rationally. Whatever the reason a person gives, if it is helping them to manage their daily stresses and strains and not causing any harm, then it should be recommended.
- Self-esteem – people will commonly report feeling better about themselves with exercise, and it is likely that this will positively impact their quality of life (Biddle et al, 2001, pp 88–117).

THE GREAT OUTDOORS

It is often claimed that exercise outdoors boosts mood and may be better for creating the feel-good factor than training indoors. This notion has certainly been taken on board by some health initiatives and exercise referral schemes across the country, with walking schemes and outdoor initiatives increasingly popular. The Green Gym provides exercise for people through involvement in local green-fingered schemes, helping with gardening or nature conservation. Similarly, the University of Exeter Medical School (2013) is researching what it has termed 'The Blue Gym', looking at an increasing amount of evidence that suggests that exercise by water has positive mental effects.

Exercise outdoors won't necessarily make any difference to the amount of calories burned or impact on weight loss, but it may well improve feelings of self-esteem, increase feelings of revitalisation and energy, decrease depression, anger, confusion, tension and other negative mood states, and importantly increase the likelihood of the person repeating the exercise session in the near future (Thompson et al, 2011).

BETTER TOGETHER

As well as outdoor activities, group-based exercise is well researched and brings favourable responses in mood for many people. The ACSM (2009) recommends that group-based sessions last 20–60 minutes at an intensity of around 50–65 per cent maximum heart rate. This low to moderate level in intensity accounts for the fact that many may be deconditioned and at greater risk of injury and dropout initially. Of course, group-based exercise may not be right for some as they may find group environments intimidating and stressful. In order to devise the most appropriate exercise routine for an individual who may be overweight, deconditioned, have low self-esteem and be anxious about exercise, make them feel at ease and work with them to identify their preferences for the following:

- Exercise environment – do they want to exercise indoors or outdoors, on their own or in groups?
- Exercise choice – what types of exercise do they feel most comfortable with? What have they done in the past that they enjoyed?

- Exercise volume and intensity – what is their current level of activity? What do the fitness assessments that you have carried out reveal?

CHILL

Relaxation is as important as exercise, and in some instances the two can be combined effectively. Mind-body exercise classes may prove very effective for stress management for some. Yoga, Pilates or Tai Chi are excellent options, with the latter being shown consistently to improve mood (Snadlund and Norlander, 2000). Tai Chi has also been shown to positively impact important physiological aspects, decreasing cortisol levels and lowering blood pressure.

Other stress-relief methods like meditation are equally useful. Breathing techniques, visualisation and muscle relaxation are all commonly used to aid stress management. The following simple technique, known as Progressive Relaxation, can be used with your clients.

- Find a quiet, comfortable place to sit.
- Sit still, eyes closed, breathe normally and focus on relaxing. Empty the mind of thoughts.
- Focus on breathing, slowly drawing air in through the nose, and out again.
- When ready, tense the calf muscles for a few seconds, then release, feeling them relax.
- Repeat this, working up through each of the muscle groups in the body to the neck and finally, face muscles.
- Take some time to reorient to the surroundings before standing.

BURNOUT

Maslach, Schaufell and Leiter (2001) describe burnout as a 'prolonged response to chronic emotional and interpersonal stressors'. In simple terms, it is a build-up of stress over time that causes negative changes in the body. One of these changes is often extreme fatigue; common in athletes training hard over long periods, or those with particularly stressful jobs. The level of fatigue these people experience means that tasks they once thought extremely simple, such as climbing the stairs, may become very challenging.

Being overweight is stressful for the body, impacting levels of insulin and other hormones, causing the body to work harder than normal. Should this be combined with other life stresses, it is possible that burnout could occur. This may include symptoms like adrenal fatigue where the adrenal glands effectively become tired and overused, subsequently being unable to produce adequate levels of adrenaline and leading to extreme tiredness.

Clients with these symptoms should be referred to medical practitioners initially and when given the all-clear to exercise should build up very gradually. Intense training, especially cardiovascular exercise should be discouraged as it will lead to fatigue quickly. Low-level, short exercise sessions should be used and progression should be very gradual, paying close attention to how the client responds during and after the session.

NUTRITION

The nutritional advice to help manage stress levels is consistent with that for weight loss.

- Eat low GI – sugary foods will cause spikes and troughs in energy levels, leading to tiredness, not useful in times of stress.
- Avoid stimulants – with stress, levels of adrenaline and cortisol rise considerably. Avoiding

foods and drinks that elevate these further can be helpful so limiting sugar, tea, and coffee may be beneficial in improving energy levels. It is not uncommon for some withdrawal symptoms to be experienced in the early stages, including headaches and cravings, but these will subside over time.

Various foods and drinks have been suggested to have a calming effect over the years. Below is a selection that clients can choose from that might help them to combat stress.

Carbohydrates are known for their mood-altering effects, and it's not just the high calorie ones that boost mood. Wholegrain or wild

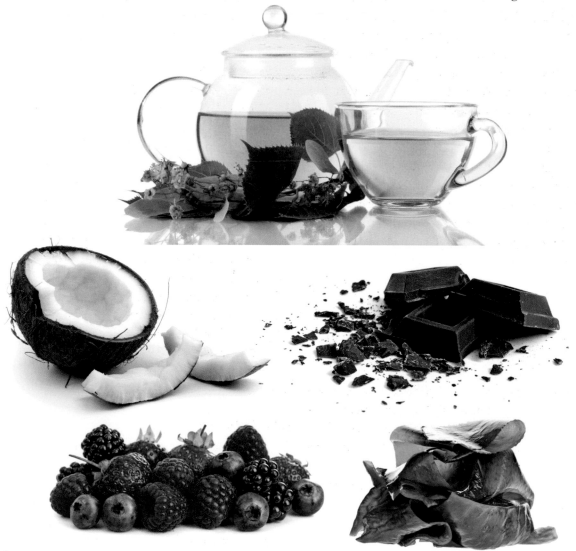

Figure 7.7 Calming food and drinks: camomile tea, coconut, dark (70 per cent cocoa solids) chocolate, berries and seaweed

rice, quinoa and oats contain tryptophan, which is converted into serotonin, known as a 'happy hormone'. Seaweed can have the same effect.

COUNSELLING

It is commonplace these days for people to have counselling in order to cope with a wide range of problems, especially stress and other mental health issues. This will be reviewed in much more detail in Chapter 8, as it is a recognised medical treatment. People may also choose to seek counselling for themselves, with methods like hypnotherapy and neurolinguistic programming (NLP), particularly popular choices.

Should clients wish to explore counselling as an option, it is important for fitness professionals to ensure they stay within the remit of their role and refer to appropriate practitioners. There will be a degree of coaching and listening as part of any fitness instructor or personal trainer's role, but if issues arise that are more about the psychological wellbeing of the client, then it is important to explain that others are better placed to support these.

SUMMARY

Lifestyle alterations are essential for successful weight loss, maintenance and health. The key messages are:

- The calorie content of alcohol may surprise some and could be the key to weight loss for many clients. As the calories in alcohol are not metabolised in the same way as foods, increased consumption can lead to greater fat stores, especially in and around the organs.
- Quitting smoking, while definitely a great idea for health, increases appetite and the risk of weight gain. This risk can be managed to an extent through the use of nicotine patches, eating low GI, and possibly by ensuring adequate chromium intake, while ensuring appropriate coping strategies are in place.
- A lack of sleep is now proven to be a risk for weight gain in both teenagers and adults. Increased ghrelin levels due to inadequate shuteye lead to higher hunger ratings.
- Stress can lead to weight gain through a variety of psychological and physiological effects. Mild stress can be effectively managed through a wide range of lifestyle changes.
- Fitness professionals can assist with lifestyle advice across all of these areas, but must ensure that they refer on to medical professionals when the client's needs are outside their scope of practice. To work with those higher risk clients referred by GPs for exercise, fitness professionals must ensure that they are suitably qualified and insured.

MEDICAL INTERVENTIONS

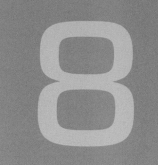

This chapter focuses primarily on the medical interventions used to help obese individuals, or those who are overweight and suffering from other medical conditions that make them high-risk for heart disease and the like. Generally these individuals should be referred into exercise programmes through their GP or other medical practitioner. Fitness professionals will require a Level 3 Exercise Referral or suitable Level 4 qualification in order to work with this group of clients, and should have the relevant insurance and first aid training.

WEIGHT LOSS SURGERY

While all overweight and obese individuals will be advised by their GP to make the dietary, exercise and lifestyle changes outlined in the previous chapters, there may be a greater urgency for some to lose weight. This may be because they have another condition; an underlying problem; are at risk of an adverse event such as a heart attack or stroke; or they may require surgery that can only be undertaken if they lose weight.

In these instances, the general advice of losing one to two pounds per week would take too long or the doctor may feel that the challenges the indi-

vidual might face, and their readiness to change mean it unlikely they would be able to achieve the desired outcome. At this point they may decide that surgery is appropriate and work with their patient to decide an appropriate course of action.

Weight loss, or bariatric surgery has been the subject of some controversy over the years, with some of the early methods used being superseded by safer and simpler ones. It has also come under the microscope because some individuals who may not actually need the surgery can travel abroad and undergo the procedure in countries subject to less regulation. There has also been some debate on the issue of individuals receiving this treatment through the NHS, when they argue that obesity is self-inflicted. In opposition to this, others have pointed out that this is also true of alcohol and smoking-related disease but that medical treatment is not denied to these people, and that the NHS was created to help everyone.

In the present day, bariatric surgery is deemed a cost-effective solution for weight loss for certain patients. Depending on the type of surgery performed, the cost of an operation may vary from £5,000–£15,000. While this may sound expensive, the instant effectiveness of the procedure compared to the costs of (often unsuccessful) lifestyle change, has made surgery the preferred option to treat obesity in the eyes of many in the medical world, as reported in the *Telegraph* (Adams, 2012).

The current NHS selection criteria for bariatric surgery are:

- A BMI of 40+
- A BMI of 35+ with at least one other medical condition that poses a risk to health (NHS Choices, 2012). Type 2 diabetes, high blood pressure and sleep apnoea are examples of such conditions.

The British Obesity Surgery Patient Association (BOSPA 2013a) identifies further criteria that a patient has to meet to be able to have surgery:

- They must be 18 or over, and possibly under 60 dependent upon the guidelines of the institution carrying out the surgery.
- They have tried and failed to lose weight previously.
- The causes for the weight gain are lifestyle-related, and the individual is aware that post-surgery they will have to commit to a substantial change in their lifestyle to maintain the effects.
- The patient is clear about the risks and benefits of the surgery and able to make an informed decision about undergoing the procedure.
- They are fit enough to undergo surgery.

TYPES OF SURGERY

There are a variety of methods available for bariatric surgery. The option chosen will depend on careful discussions between the patient and their medical practitioner, and will consider their needs, the desired outcomes and the associated risks. Even today, surgery brings with it a range of risks to be considered alongside the benefits. Surgery can lead to a range of complications due to its invasive nature, and even now the risk of death when having a gastric band fitted is 1 in 2,000, and for gastric bypass surgery it is 1 in 100 (NHS, 2013). These odds should highlight the seriousness with which the operations are treated.

Surgery can be broadly divided into two types:

- Malabsorptive
- Restrictive

Malabsorptive surgery involves any form of operation that, as its name suggests, decreases the natural ability of the body to absorb food. The main goal, of course, is to decrease the amount of calories absorbed, although careful consideration is taken to ensure that post-surgery the patient is able to take on the required amounts of vitamins, minerals and other nutrients their body requires, while at the same time losing weight.

Restrictive surgery, rather than decreasing the ability of the body to absorb foods, prevents it being taken on in the first place. The surgical procedure is generally designed to restrict the size of the stomach and this, in turn, decreases the amount of food the patient can consume before feeling full. The various surgical methods used in both types of procedure are listed in the table below, and some of the more common methods are described in detail afterwards.

GASTRIC BYPASS

The human intestines are extremely efficient at absorbing energy and nutrients from the food

Table 8.1	Identifying common weight loss surgery procedures	
Malabsorptive procedures	**Restrictive procedures**	
• Biliopancreatic diversion* • Duodenal switch* * *Commonly referred to as gastric bypass operations*	• Stomach stapling (vertical banded gastroplasty) • Sleeve gastrectomy • Gastric band (laproscopic gastroplasty)	

we consume. The various components of the system, including the small intestine, large intestine, duodenum and jejunum all have their part to play in ensuring this efficiency. In fact, the small intestines, if laid out flat, would stretch for around seven to ten metres. It is the length of these organs, and the structure of their walls that enables so much of the food eaten to be absorbed.

Bypass operations aim to limit the ability of the body to absorb food by diverting it away from specific parts of the digestive system, in much the same way that a road bypass diverts traffic away from busy areas. A duodenal switch is one such procedure. Here much of the stomach is removed and this is then attached to the final section of small intestine, missing out large portions of this organ and limiting the amount of energy that can be absorbed.

STOMACH STAPLING

No longer routinely used, stomach stapling was a restrictive procedure. This involved the stapling of part of the stomach, combined with the application of a band, making it smaller and quickly leading to discomfort should the patient try to eat

too much. However, issues included the staples tearing away and the dramatic reduction in stomach size leading to discomfort and even vomiting for some when they ate.

GASTRIC BAND

Known in the medical world as laparoscopic gastroplasty, gastric banding involves the insertion of a band around the stomach. This again makes the area of the stomach smaller, reducing the amount of food and, therefore, calories that the patient can consume. Bands are adjustable dependent on patient progress, and it is possible that the patient may have the band removed at a later stage once they have achieved their goal weight. In many cases it is left in place, both to prevent them from relapsing back to previous behaviours and because the risks of carrying out further surgery may not outweigh the benefits. It is possible for people to lose over 50 per cent of their excess weight with this form of surgery (BOSPA, 2013b).

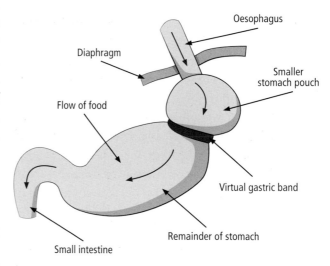

Figure 8.1 How a gastric band works

GASTRIC SLEEVE

This involves the removal of part of the stomach, again making the area available to receive food smaller and decreasing the amount that can be taken in.

SURGERY AND THE FITNESS PROFESSIONAL

After surgery, individuals will be encouraged to make lifestyle changes to support their weight loss and long-term maintenance. They will be given specific guidelines by their surgeon or medical practitioner regarding the foods they can consume and the activity they should take part in.

Surgeons may recommend very low-calorie diets in the immediate run-up to an operation, often very low in carbohydrate so as to decrease glycogen stores and decrease the size of the liver. This increases the chances of carrying out surgery without having to make large incisions as technology these days allows for the use of small instruments and tiny cameras for operations.

Post-surgery patients are given diet guidelines immediately after the operation. Straight after surgery food has to be very easily digestible and so is mashed up. Portion sizes are smaller and people are advised to stay well hydrated and to stop eating when full. Over time they can progress back to solid foods but still have to follow a restricted calorie diet and eat healthy options. It is recommended that they do not consume sugary drinks as these can pass through the new smaller stomach very quickly, leading to high calorie intake and making it difficult to lose weight.

The British Obesity Surgery Patient Association (BOSPA, 2013c) state that some foods remain problematic for patients after their operation due to their size, shape or texture. These include broccoli, pineapple, dried fruit, nuts and meat. They recommend that foods are finely chopped or mashed to enable easier digestion. As an exercise professional you should work with the patient and their medical practitioner/dietician to ensure they follow the guidelines.

Exercise guidance is fairly generic and recommends increases in lifestyle activities and referral by GPs into recognised schemes. As an instructor it will be important to consider the following when designing programmes:

- Reduced perceived energy levels with lower calorie intake in the initial phase.
- Discomfort in the weeks after surgery. It is unwise to begin exercise until this has settled down.
- Any specific advice given by the surgeon or GP.
- The need to send the patient to their doctor straight away should any issues or signs and symptoms of complications arise.

MEDICATIONS

The search for the 'magic bullet', a pill that helps bring about effective, permanent weight loss, has been considered the holy grail of the pharmaceutical industry for many years. To date this has not been discovered and it is unlikely that it will be, especially in light of the complex interplay of risk factors that lead to obesity.

A number of medications have been proposed or prescribed for the treatment of obesity over the years; however at present the National Institute for Health and Clinical Excellence (NICE, 2006) only recommends one for use in the UK. This is known as Orlistat.

Orlistat

The drug treatment of choice at present, Orlistat, also known as Xenical, works by decreasing the absorption of the fat a person eats. Instead of being absorbed it is passed out in the stool. This can lead to unpleasant side effects for people, as the stool will be loose and oily due to the presence of a large amount of fat, meaning they may need frequent toilet visits. Many taking this medication will say that because of these unpleasant side effects, they are less likely to eat fatty foods, so Orlistat acts more as a deterrent than anything.

In recent years, Orlistat, under the trade name Alli, has controversially been made available for people to buy online or over the counter without prescription. It is not recommended unless a person has a BMI of greater than 28, but many have argued that being mildly overweight should be managed through lifestyle change and that the ability to purchase online mean that sales are hard to monitor safely and effectively.

If a client has been prescribed Orlistat, there may be some important things to consider when planning and delivering exercise sessions and lifestyle changes with them:

- Ask if there are any exercises that aggravate their stomach. This may include higher impact cardio-vascular activities, but can be unique to the individual.
- Consider the location and accessibility of toilets when planning exercise.
- Be aware that many may be uncomfortable discussing these effects, and that suffering an incident while exercising may have a big impact on self-esteem and comfort in the exercise environment.
- Agree dietary changes with your client taking into account the effects of the medication.

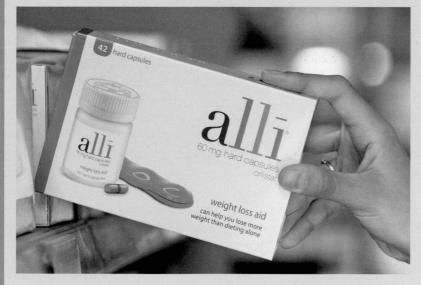

Figure 8.2 Alli – the over-the-counter pill for weight loss

NOT SO NICE

In recent years, a medication known as Sibutramine has had the National Institute for Health and Clinical Excellence (NICE) recommendation for use withdrawn, due to evidence that showed a markedly increased risk of clotting and strokes (US Food and Drug Administration, 2010). NICE regulate all the treatments and practices, including medications, provided by the National Health Service.

Various medications have been either withdrawn or rejected for use in the UK over the years, although some are still used elsewhere around the world. A number of these have assisted weight loss by speeding up metabolic rate, increasing the calorie burn of those using them. This stimulant effect, while certainly proven to work, has many risks associated with it, including, but not limited to, increased heart rate and blood pressure, tremors and blood sugar fluctuations.

But it's not just medications that can be problematic. Type 'weight loss tablets' into any Internet search engine these days and you'll be greeted with an overwhelming number of search returns, all offering the ability to buy 'natural' or 'herbal' supplements that help people to achieve their weight loss dreams. Most will come with 'proven' or 'guaranteed to work' marketing slogans, but at best most will be ineffective, not based on any scientific proof, and at worst they could be dangerous and increase the risk of health problems. As fitness professionals, if you discover that a client is taking any of these you should cease exercise sessions and advise them to visit their GP to discuss the matter. The GP should then inform you of the course of action they have recommended and whether or not the client is safe to begin exercise again.

PILLS FOR ILLS

Obese clients will often have a range of other conditions (known as comorbidities). Fitness professionals suitably qualified to work with these clients (Exercise Referral or Level 4 Specialist) should be aware of the range of medications that they may be taking and the effects these could have on their responses to exercise. Table 8.2 identifies a range of very common medications that clients may be prescribed. To find out about others, ask a medical practitioner or log on to and register with the British National Formulary (www.bnf.org.uk). This organisation lists all current medications available for prescription in the UK, providing details on how they work and potential side effects that may impact exercise sessions.

Some overweight or obese clients may also be taking medication for bone or joint problems. If these have a painkilling effect, this should be considered when checking the intensity of sessions. Clients with sleep apnoea may use oxygen therapy in their sleep and while this should not directly affect exercise sessions, instructors should be aware that these clients are often severely deconditioned, and should start with low volume and intensity. Before every session, checks should be made to ensure clients are taking medications and that no new signs or symptoms have presented themselves. If a client is not taking their medication as instructed, or their condition has changed, exercise should be suspended and they should be signposted to their medical practitioner. Exercise should only recommence when the medical practitioner says that it is safe to do so.

Table 8.2	Guide to common medications	
Medication	**How it works**	**Possible side effects**
Biguanides, e.g. metformin	Increases sensitivity to insulin in type 2 diabetics	Nausea, diarrhoea and abdominal pain. Lactic acidosis – this can be severe so send back to GP instantly if client informs you of unusual tiredness, dizziness, confusion or difficulty breathing.
Insulin	Used for type 1 diabetics, or type 2 diabetics with severe symptoms, insulin injections act to replace the insulin that the body no longer produces. It helps to lower blood sugar levels.	Incorrect dosage/timing may lead to hypoglycaemia. Failure to take may lead to hyperglycaemia.
Beta blockers, e.g. atenolol	Blocks the action of adrenaline to lower blood pressure in those with hypertension.	Heart rate will be lowered and unlikely to rise above 130–140 bpm. RPE scales are preferred to monitor intensity.
ACE Inhibitors, e.g. lisinopril	Inhibit the action of Angiotensin Converting Enzymes	Low blood pressure may make clients dizzy, especially if moving from seated to standing exercises. Stomach problems can also occur.
Statins, e.g. simvastatin	Lowers the ability of the body to produce cholesterol, decreasing LDL cholesterol levels by 20–60 per cent.	Muscle wastage and soreness may affect strength and endurance, decreasing duration and intensity of sessions.
Antidepressants, e.g. tricyclic antidepressants or selective serotonin reuptake inhibitors (SSRIs)	Alter levels of neurotransmitters linked with mood.	A wide variety of symptoms are possible that may impact exercise. These include: • Changes in energy levels • Decreased awareness • Changes in mood • Changes in heart rate • Visual problems • Dizziness and hypotension • Changes in weight

COUNSELLING

For some people, a medical practitioner may also recommend that they undergo counselling to help with their weight loss, although this is not currently listed as a treatment option for obesity on the NHS website. This may be because they have underlying issues with food, or low self-esteem linked to psychological trauma or a medical condition linked to their weight gain. It is not uncommon for those with a condition who are obese to also be suffering from depression and this may be the reason for referral to a counsellor.

There are various forms of counselling, but two commonly used by the NHS are cognitive behavioural therapy (CBT) and psychotherapy.

COGNITIVE BEHAVIOURAL THERAPY

CBT uses conversation to help people to change thoughts (cognitive) and the things they do (behaviour). It looks at taking problems and dividing them into more manageable chunks. CBT has been examined in studies for the treatment of binge eating and for weight management in general with mixed results (Grilo and Masheb, 2005; Rapoport et al, 2000).

PSYCHOTHERAPY

Often used in the treatment of depression, it can be done individually, with families or in groups. Again it involves talking about problems and working through them in an attempt to find solutions. CBT is a specific form of psychotherapy.

SUMMARY

- Weight loss surgery may be recommended for extremely obese individuals or those with other conditions that increase their risk of complications. It can be effective for weight loss, although there are risks.
- Post-surgery, if suitably qualified, exercise professionals may be asked to support lifestyle change by designing safe exercise programmes. These should be low intensity and take into account any recommendations by the surgeon.
- Orlistat is the only recommended drug treatment for obesity in the UK at present. It can also be bought over the counter as Alli. Fitness professionals should be aware of the potentially uncomfortable side effects of this medication for their clients.
- Obese clients who also have comorbidities may take a wide range of medications. Instructors need to be aware of the implications of these for exercise.
- Therapy may be used by GPs for treatment of those with depression where obesity is a secondary factor.

ACKNOWLEDGEMENTS

I have spent all of my working life in the fitness industry, and it is more than a job to me, it is my hobby, my passion and a large part of who I am. I wanted to write this book so that in some way I may be able to contribute to making the world a happier, healthier place. I hope that you take something from it that can help you or your clients.

There are many people that I would like to thank for helping me get to a point where this was possible. They are:

- My family, in particular my parents Bill and Jude, and sister Suzi for always believing in me, never questioning my decision to change my career path or up sticks, and for offering me endless support in more ways than you will ever know.
- My partner Vicky for putting up with me spending hours in front of my computer and for being rational when I was stressing about deadlines. A massive thank you also for your excellent review of the current diets that people use in their attempts to lose weight.
- Every tutor, personal trainer, fitness instructor, physiologist and member of the fitness and education community I have ever had the pleasure to work with. I have learned so much from you all and have enjoyed every minute. In particular on this book my thanks to Chris Foster for his eagle eye and to Simon Toseland for his much appreciated advice on structure, layout and feel of the book. Also to everyone I have worked with at Lifetime Training for your help in constantly striving to learn new things and make fitness education better.
- Every learner that has ever attended one of my courses. I think I have learned more from you than you from me.
- All of my clients who I have had the pleasure to work with over the years. Thank you for your honesty and hard work, and for teaching me what to do and what not to do to help you reach your goals. Courses and books taught me many things, but I learned much more when I had to apply it in the real world.

RESOURCES

The following is a useful list of charities, websites and organisations that provide research, information and education on obesity and related conditions, health and exercise.

Alcoholics Anonymous –
www.alcoholics-anonymous.org.uk
American Journal of Clinical Nutrition –
ajcn.nutrition.org
Association for the Study of Obesity –
www.aso.org.uk
Australian and New Zealand Obesity Society –
www.anzos.com
Australian Institute of Health and Welfare –
www.aihw.gov.au/overweight-and-obesity/
Australian National Health and Medical
Research Council – www.nhmrc.gov.au/
your-health/obesity-and-overweight
Balance Weight Loss –
www.balanceweightloss.co.uk
British Heart Foundation –
www.bhf.org.uk
British National Formulary –
www.bnf.org
British Nutrition Foundation –
www.nutrition.org.uk
Department of Health – www.gov.uk/
government/organisations/department-of-health
Diabetes UK – www.diabetes.org.uk
ExRx: Exercise Prescription –
www.exrx.net

International Association for the Study of
Obesity – www.iaso.org
International Diabetes Federation –
www.idf.org
International Journal of Obesity –
www.nature.com/ijo/index.html
International Obesity Taskforce –
www.iaso.org/iotf/
MEND – www.mendcentral.org
MIND – www.mind.org.uk
National Institute for Health and Clinical Excellence – www.nice.org.uk/guidance/cg43
National Obesity Forum –
www.nationalobesityforum.org.uk
National Sleep Foundation –
www.sleepfoundation.org
NHS Quit Smoking – smokefree.nhs.uk
Obesity Action Campaign –
www.obesityac.org/charity-launched-
to-address-obesity-epidemic
Obesity Action Coalition –
www.obesityaction.org
Obesity Australia –
www.obesityaustralia.org
Obesity Journal – www.obesity.org/
publications/obesity-journal.htm
Obesity Society – www.obesity.org
Shape up America – www.shapeup.org
US Department of Agriculture – www.usda.gov/
wps/portal/usda/usdahome
World Health Organization –
www.who.int/topics/obesity/en/

REFERENCES

PREFACE

NHS Choices (26th August, 2011) 'Half of UK obese by 2030'. www.nhs.uk/news/2011/08August/Pages/half-of-uk-predicted-to-be-obese-by-2030.aspx, accessed 01/05/13.

Public Health England (2013) 'About obesity: UK prevalence and trends'. www.noo.org.uk/NOO_about_obesity/adult_obesity/UK_prevalence_and_trends, accessed 01/05/13.

US Center for Disease Control and Prevention (2011) 'Adult obesity facts'. www.cdc.gov/obesity/data/adult.html, accessed 19/12/13.

CHAPTER 1

Atkinson, R.L. (2007) 'Viruses as an etiology of obesity', *Mayo Clinic Proceedings*, 82 (10), 1192–1198.

Centers for Disease Control and Prevention (May 17th, 2013) 'Genomics and health: genes and obesity'. www.cdc.gov/genomics/resources/diseases/obesity/obesedit.htm, accessed 10/07/13.

Department of Health (September, 2011) 'Obesity: general information' webarchive.nationalarchives.gov.uk/20130107105354/www.dh.gov.uk/en/Publichealth/Obesity/DH_078098, accessed 10/10/13.

Diabetes Prevention Program Research Group (2002) 'The Diabetes Prevention Program (DPP)', *Diabetes Care*, 25 (12), 2165–2171.

Duncan, S.H., Lobley, G.E., Holtrop, G., Ince, J., Johnstone, A.M., Louis, P. and Flint, J. (2008) 'Human colonic microbiota associated with diet, obesity and weight loss', *International Journal of Obesity*, 32, 1720–1724.

Eckel, R. (1997) 'Obesity and heart disease: a statement for healthcare professionals from the Nutrition Committee, American Heart Association', *Circulation*, 96, 3248–3250.

Hall, J. (1st February, 2012) 'Britons are biggest online shoppers in developed world', *The Telegraph*, www.telegraph.co.uk/news/uknews/9054400/Britons-are-biggest-online-shoppers-in-developed-world.html, accessed 10/10/13.

Harvard School of Public Health (2013) 'The obesity prevention source: ethnic differences in BMI and disease'. www.hsph.harvard.edu/obesity-prevention-source/ethnic-differences-in-bmi-and-disease-risk/, accessed 15/07/13.

Jialal, I., Devaraj, S., Kaur, H., Adams-Huet, B. and Bremner, A.A. (2013) 'Increased chemerin and decreased omentin-1 in both adipose tissue and plasma in nascent metabolic syndrome', *Journal of Endocrinology & Metabolism*, 98 (3).

Mail Online (20th September, 2013) 'Obese two-year-old Saudi Arabian boy is the world's youngest person to have gastric bypass surgery'. http://www.dailymail.co.uk/news/article-2426722/Saudi-Arabian-boys-gastric-bypass-surgery-worlds-youngest-2-years-old.html, accessed 10/10/13.

Mohs, M.E., Watson, R.R. and Leonard-Green, T. (1990) 'Nutritional effects of marijuana, heroin, cocaine and nicotine', *Journal of the American Dietetic Association*, 90 (9), 1261–1267.

Mendes, E. (2011) 'In US, self-reported weight up nearly 20 pounds since 1990'. www.gallup.com/poll/150947/self-reported-weight-nearly-pounds-1990.aspx, accessed 19/12/13.

National Cancer Institute (2012) 'Obesity and cancer risk'. www.cancer.gov/cancertopics/factsheet/Risk/obesity, accessed 07/10/13.

NHS Choices (2012) '10 health benefits of stopping smoking'. www.nhs.uk/Livewell/smoking/Pages/Betterlives.aspx, accessed 20/12/13.

Ong, K.K. and Loos, R.J.F. (2007) 'Rapid infancy weight gain and subsequent obesity: systematic reviews and hopeful suggestions', *Acta Paediatrica*, 95 (8), 904–908.

Ready, R. and Burton, K. (2010) *Neuro-linguistc programming for dummies,* 2nd edition. John Wiley & Sons, Ltd, England.

Scheinbach, S. (1998) 'Probiotics: functionality and commercial status', Biotechnology Advances, 16 (3), 581–608.

Spiegel, K., Taslai, E., Penev, P. and Van Cauter, E. (2004) 'Brief communication: sleep curtailment in healthy young men is associated with decreased leptin levels, elevated ghrelin levels, and increased hunger and appetite', *Annals of Internal Medicine*, 141 (11).

Taheri, S., Lin, L., Austin, D., Young, T. and Mignot, E. (2004) 'Short sleep duration is associated with reduced leptin, elevated ghrelin, and increased Body Mass Index', *PLoS Medicine*, 1 (3) e62.

Turnbaugh, P.J., Ley, R.E., Mahowald, M.A., Magrini, V., Mardis, E.R and Gordon, J.I. (2006) 'An obesity-associated gut microbiome with increased capacity for energy harvest', *Nature*, 444, 1027–1031.

Vasilakopoulou, A. and le Roux, C.W. (2007) 'Could a virus contribute to weight gain?' *International Journal of Obesity*, 31, 1350-1356.

CHAPTER 2

Amigo, I. and Fernandez, C. (2007) 'Effects of diets and their role in weight control', *Psychology, Health and Medicine*, 12 (3), 321-327.

Centers for Disease Control and Prevention (May 17th, 2013) 'Genomics and health: genes and obesity'. www.cdc.gov/genomics/resources/diseases/obesity/obesedit.htm, accessed 10/07/13.

Drapeau, V., Thierren, F., Richard, D. and Tremblay, A. (2003) 'Is visceral obesity a physiological adaptation to stress?' *Panminerva Medical*, 45–195.

Epstein, L.H., Temple, J.L., Neaderhiser, B.J., Salis, R.J., Erbe, R.W. and Leddy, J.J. (2007) 'Food reinforcement, the dopamine D receptor genotype, and energy intake in obese and nonobese humans', *Behavioural Neuroscience*, 121 (5), 877–886.

Guldbrand, H., Dizdar, B., Bunjaku, T., Lindstrom, M., Bachrach-Lindstrom, M., Fredrikson, M., Ostgren, C.J. and Nystrom, F.H. (2012) 'In type 2 diabetes, randomisation to advice to follow a low-carbohydrate diet transiently improves glycaemic control compared with advice to follow a low-fat diet producing a similar weight loss', *Diabetologia*, 55 (8), 2118–2127.

Kivimaki, M., Head, J., Ferrie, J.E., Shipley, M.J., Brunner, E., Vahtera, J. and Marmot, M. (2006) 'Work stress, weight gain and weight loss:

evidence for bidirectional effects of job strain on body mass index in the Whitehall II study', *International Journal of Obesity*, 30, 982–987.

Marshall, J.A. and Bessesen, D.H. (2002) 'Dietary fat and the development of type 2 diabetes', *Diabetes Care*, 25 (3), 620–622.

McArdle, W.D., Katch, F.I. and Katch, V.L. (2010) *Exercise physiology: nutrition, energy and human performance* 7th edition, Lippincott, Williams & Wilkins, USA.

Müller, M.J., Bosy-Westphal, A. and Hemsfeld, S.B. (2010) 'Is there evidence for a set point that regulates human body weight?' *F1000 Medicine Reports*, 2, 59.

Myers, M.G., Cowley, M.A. and Munzberg, H. (2008) 'Mechanics of leptin action and leptin resistance', *Annual Review of Physiology*, 70, 537–556.

Pereira, M.A., Swain, J., Goldfine, A.B., Rifai, N. and Ludwig, D.S. (2004) 'Effects of a low-glycemic load diet on resting energy expenditure and heart disease risk factors during weight loss', *Journal of the American Medical Association*, 292 (20), 2482–2490.

Ravussin, E. and Bogardus, C. (2000) 'Energy balance and weight regulation: genetics versus environment', *British Journal of Nutrition*, 83, Supplement 1, S17–S20.

Starke, A.A., Erhardt, G., Berger, M. and Zimmermann, H. (1984) 'Elevated pancreatic glucagon in obesity', *Diabetes*, 33 (3), 277–280.

Taubes, G. (25th April, 2013) 'Are we ignoring the true cause of obesity?' *Business Insider*, www.businessinsider.com/carbohydrates-insulin-and-obesity-2013-4, accessed 25/04/13.

Thyroid UK (2010) 'Hypothyroidism'. www.thyroiduk.org.uk/tuk/about_the_thyroid/hypothyroidism.html, accessed 22/12/13.

Torres, S. (2007) 'Relationship between stress, eating behaviour, and obesity', *Nutrition*, 23 (11), 887–894.

Weinsier, R.L., Nagy, T.R., Hunter, G.R., Darnell, B.E., Hensrdu, D.D. and Weiss, H.L. (2000) 'Do adaptive changes in metabolic rate favor weight regain in weight-reduced individuals? An examination of the set-point theory', *American Journal of Clinical Nutrition*, 72 (5), 1088–1094.

Wing, R.R. and Phelan, S. (2005) 'Long-term weight loss maintenance', *The American Journal of Clinical Nutrition*, 82 (1), 2225-2255.

Wurtman, J.J. and Frusztajer, N.T. (2009) *The Serotonin Power Diet*. Rodale Books, USA.

CHAPTER 3

Borg G.A.V. (1998) 'Rating of Perceived Exertion and Pain Scales'.: *Human Kinetics*, Champaign, IL.

Bray, G.A. and Gray, D.S. (1988) 'Obesity: Part 1 – Pathogenesis', *Western Journal of Medicine*, 149 (4), 429–441.

Castaneda, C., Layne, J.E., Munoz-Orians, L., Gordon, P.L., Walsmith, J., Foldvari, M., Roubenoff, R., Tucker, K.L. and Nelson, M.E. (2002) 'A randomized controlled trial of resistance exercise training to improve glycemic control in older adults with type 2 diabetes', *Diabetes*, 25, 2335-2341.

Centre for Disease Control and Prevention (2013) 'The 30-second chair stand test'. www.cdc.gov/homeandrecreationalsafety/pdf/steadi/30_second_chair_stand_test.pdf, accessed 01/10/13.

Deurenberg-Yap, M. and Chew, S.K. (2002) 'Elevated body fat percentage and cardiovascular risks at low Body Mass Index levels among Singaporean Chinese, Malays and Indians', *Obesity Reviews*, 3 (3), 209–215.

Eknoyan, G. (2008) 'Adolphe Quetelet (1796–1874) – the average man and indices of obesity', *Nephrology Dialysis Transplantation*, 23, 47–51.

ExRx.net (2013) www.exrx.net/Testing/Skinfold-Procedures.html, accessed 21/05/13.

Ferreira, I., Snijder, M.B., Twisk, J.W.R., van Mechelen, W., Kemper, H.C.G., Seidell, J.C. and Stehouwer, C.D.A. (2004) 'Central fat mass versus peripheral fat and lean mass: opposite (adverse versus favorable) associations with arterial stiffness? The Amsterdam Growth and Health Longitudinal Study', *The Journal of Clinical Endocrinology & Metabolism*, 89 (6), 2632–2639.

Golden, C. (January 16th, 2013) 'Being pear-shaped carries health risks too, say researchers'. www.davisenterprise.com/local-news/ucd/being-pear-shaped-carries-health-risks-too-researchers-say/, accessed 10/07/13.

Harvard School of Public Health (2013) 'The obesity prevention source: ethnic differences in BMI and disease risk'. www.hsph.harvard.edu/obesity-prevention-source/ethnic-differences-in-bmi-and-disease-risk/, accessed 27/07/13.

International Diabetes Federation (2007) 'Criteria of metabolic syndrome in children and adults'. www.idf.org/metabolic-syndrome/children/criteria, accessed 06/06/13.

Jackson, A.S. and Pollock, M. (1985) 'Practical assessment of body composition', *Physician and Sports Medicine*, 13, 76-90.

Jones C.J. and Rikli R.E. (2002) 'Measuring functional fitness of older adults', *The Journal on Active Aging*, March/April, 4–30.

Krishan, K and Vij, K (2007) 'Diurnal variation of stature in three adults and one child', *Anthropologist*, 9(2): 113–117

McArdle, W.D, Katch, F.I. and Katch, V.L. (2010) *Exercise Physiology: Nutrition, Energy and Human Performance*, 7th edition, Lipincott, Williams & Wilkins, USA.

Merriam-Webster Online Dictionary (2013) Rapport. www.merriam-webster.com/dictionary/rapport, accessed 21/05/13.

NHS Choices (2012) 'Why is my waist size important?' www.nhs.uk/chq/Pages/849.aspx?CategoryID=51, accessed 06/06/13.

NHS Choices (24th August, 2013) 'Why body shape matters'. www.nhs.uk/Livewell/loseweight/Pages/Appleorpear.aspx, accessed 01/10/13.

Oppliger, R.A., Looney, M.A. and Tipton, C.M. (1987) 'Reliability of hydrostatic weighing and skinfold measurements of body composition using a generalisability study', *Human Biology*, 59 (1), 77–96.

Ross R., Goodpaster B., Kelley D. and Boada F. (2000) 'Magnetic resonance imaging in human body composition research. From quantitative to qualitative tissue measurement', *Annals of the New York Academy of Science*, 904, 12–17.

Sibella, F., Galli. M., Romei, M., Montesano, A. and Crivellini, M. (2003) 'Biomechanical analysis of sit-to-stand movement in normal and obese subjects', *Clinical Biomechanics*, 18 (8), 745–750.

Towfighi A, Zheng L, Ovbiagele B. (2009) 'Sex-specific trends in midlife coronary heart disease risk and prevalence', *Archives of Internal Medicine*, 169, 1762–1766.

Wolfe, R.R. (2006) 'The underappreciated role of muscle in health and disease', *The American Journal of Clinical Nutrition*, 84 (3), 475–482.

World Health Organization (2006) 'BMI classification', http://apps.who.int/bmi/index.jsp?introPage=intro_3.html, accessed 26/07/13.

World Health Organization (2008) 'Waist circumference and waist-to-hip ratio: report of a WHO expert consultation', Geneva 8–11th December 2008.

CHAPTER 4

Drach-Zahavy, A. and Erez, M. (2002). 'Challenge versus threat effects on the goal-performance relationship', *Organizational Behaviour and Human Performance*, 88, 667–682.

Fishbach, A., Eyal, T. and Finkelstein, A.R. (2010) 'How positive and negative feedback motivate goal pursuit', *Social and Personality Psychology*, 4 (8), 517–530.

House, J.S. (1987) 'Social support and social structure', *Sociological Forum*, 2 (1), 135–146.

Johnson, S. S., Paiva, A. L., Cummins, C. O., Johnson, J. L., Dyment, S. J., Wright, J. A., Prochaska, J. O., Prochaska, J. M. and Sherman, K. (2008). 'Trans-theoretical model-based multiple behaviour intervention for weight management: effectiveness on a population basis', *Preventive Medicine*, 46, 238–246.

Locke, E.A and Latham, G.P (2006) 'New directions in goal-setting theory', *Current Directions in Psychological Science*, 15 (5), 265–268.

NICE (October, 2007) 'Behaviour change: NICE Public Health Guidance 6'. www.nice.org.uk/nicemedia/live/11868/37987/37987.pdf, accessed 10/08/13.

Olson, A.L and Edelstein, E. (1968) 'Spot reduction of subcutaneous adipose tissue', *Research Quarterly: American Association for Health, Physical Education and Recreation*, 39 (3), 647–652.

Poliquin, C. (2013), 'The Poliquin Biosignature Modulation'. www.poliquingroup.com/Education/Biosignature.aspx, accessed 23/10/13.

Prochaska, J.O and DiClemente, C.C. (1984) *The transtheoretical approach: crossing traditional boundaries of therapy*. Dow Jones-Irwin Illinois, USA.

Schwartzer, R. (2013) 'The health action process approach', Freie University, Berlin, userpage.fu-berlin.de/health/hapa.htm, accessed 01/09/13.

Tuah, N., Amiel, C., Qureshi, S., Car, J., Kaur, B. and Majeed, A. (2011) 'Trans-theoretical model for dietary and physical exercise modification in weight loss management for overweight and obese adults', *Cochrane Database Systematic Reviews*. 5;10:CD008066.pub2. PMID 21975777, accessed 20/08/13.

Uchino, B. (2006) 'Social support and health: a review of physiological processes potentially underlying links to disease outcomes', *Journal of Behavioural Medicine*, 29, 377–387.

Weinsier, R.L, Wilson, L.J. and Lee, J. (1995), 'Medically safe rate of weight loss for the treatment of obesity: a guideline based on risk of gallstone formation', *The American Journal of Medicine*, 98 (2), 115–117.

Wing, R.R. and Phelan, S. (2005) 'Long-term weight loss maintenance', *The American Journal of Clinical Nutrition*, 82 (1), 2225–2255.

CHAPTER 5

ACSM (2011) 'ACSM information on … selecting and effectively using hydration for fitness'. www.acsm.org/docs/brochures/selecting-and-effectively-using-hydration-for-fitness.pdf, accessed 11/08/13.

Anderson, R.A. (2000) 'Chromium in the prevention and control of diabetes', *Diabetes and Metabolism*, 26, 22–27.

Andrade, A.M., Greene, G.W. and Melanson, K.J. (2008) 'Eating slowly led to decreases in energy intake within meals in healthy women', *Journal of the American Dietetic Association*, 108 (7), 1186–1191.

Apovian, C.M. (2004) 'Sugar-sweetened soft-drinks, obesity, and type 2 diabetes', *The Journal of the American Medical Association*, 292 (8), 978–979.

Appleton, K. and Rogers, P.J. (2004) 'Food and mood', *Women's Health Medicine*, 1 (1), 4–6.

Astrup, A., Larsen, T.M. and Harper, A. (2004) 'Atkins and other low-carbohydrate diets: hoax or an effective tool for weight loss?' *The Lancet*, 364 (9437), 897–899.

BBC News (23rd October, 2013) 'Saturated fat heart disease "myth"'. www.bbc.co.uk/news/health-24625808, accessed 23/10/13.

Beimers, E. (2012) 'Food and mood: The relationship between food and mood disorders from a neurobiological perspective: the role of tryptophan'. arno.uvt.nl/show.cgi?fid=127219, accessed 17/09/13.

Blau, J.N., Kell, C.A. and Sperling, J.M. (2004) 'Water deprivation headache: a new headache with two variants', *Headache: The Journal of Head and Face Pain*, 44 (1), 79–83.

Boseley, S. (7th September, 2013) 'Smoothies and fruit juices are a new risk to health, US scientists warn'. *The Guardian*, www.theguardian.com/society/2013/sep/07/smoothies-fruit-juices-new-health-risk, accessed 07/09/13.

British Nutrition Foundation (2012) 'Protein'. www.nutrition.org.uk/nutritionscience/nutrients/protein, accessed 03/07/13.

Connor, S. (2013) 'Fat chance of slimming: dieters who eat high-fibre foods consume more calories, scientists say'. *The Independent* Online, 18th February, 2013. www.independent.co.uk/news/science/fat-chance-of-slimming-dieters-who-eat-highfibre-foods-consume-more-calories-scientists-say-8500122.html, viewed June 2013.

Crown Copyright (2013) 'The eatwell plate'. www.nhs.uk/Livewell/Goodfood/Documents/Eatwellplate.pdf, accessed 27/10/13.

Davy, B.M., Dennis, E.A., Dengo, A.L., Wilson, K.L. and Davy, K.P. (2008) 'Water consumption reduces energy intake at a breakfast meal in obese older adults', *Journal of the American Dietetic Association*, 108 (7), 236–1239.

Dunn, R. (2013) 'Science reveals why calorie counts are all wrong', *The Scientific American*, 16th September, 2013.

Eisenstein, J., Roberts, S.B., Dallal, G. and Saltzman, E. (2002) 'High-protein weight-loss diets: are they safe and do they work? A review of the experimental and epidemiologic data', *Nutrition Reviews*, 60 (7), 189–200.

Fletcher, R.H. and Fairfield, K.M. (2002) 'Vitamins for chronic disease prevention in adults', *The Journal of the American Medical Association*, 287 (23), 3153–3154

Friedman, A. (2004) 'High-protein diets: potential effects on the kidney in renal health and disease', *American Journal of Kidney Diseases*, 54 (6), 950–962.

Genschow, O., Reutner, L. and Wänke, M. (2012) 'The colour red reduces snack food and soft drink intake', *Appetite*, 58 (2), 699–702.

Gov.UK (19th June, 2013) Press release: 'Final design of consistent nutritional labelling system given green light'. www.gov.uk/government/

news/final-design-of-consistent-nutritional-labelling-system-given-green-light, accessed 29/12/13.

Halton, T.L and Hu, F. (2004) 'The effects of high protein diets on thermogenesis, satiety and weight loss: a critical review', *Journal of the American College of Nutrition*, 23 (5), 373–385.

Judelson, D.A., Maresh, C.M., Anderson, J.M., Armstrong, L.E., Casa, D.J., Kraemer, W.J. and Volek, J.S. (2007) 'Hydration and muscular performance', *Sports Medicine*, 37 (10), 907–921.

Lichtman, S.W., Pisarska, K., Berman, E.R., Pestone, M., Dowling, H., Offenbacher, E., Weisel, H., Heshka, S., Matthews, D.E. and Heymsfield, S.B. (1992) 'Discrepancy between self-reported and actual caloric intake and exercise in obese subjects', *The New England Journal of Medicine*, 327 (27), 1893–1898.

Ludwig, S. (2000) 'Symposium: dietary composition and obesity: do we need to look beyond dietary fat? Dietary Glycemic Index and obesity', *American Journal of Clinical Nutrition*, 130, 280s–283s.

McKenna, P. (2005) *I can make you thin*. Bantam Press, London, UK.

Mail Online (2009) www.dailymail.co.uk/news/article-1227743/Its-official--eat-stay-healthy.html, accessed 02/08/13.

McFerran, B. (2013) 'Lay theories of obesity predict actual body mass', *Psychological Science*, 24 (8), 1428–1436.

Miller, W.C., Koceja, D.M. and Hamilton, E.J. (1997) 'A meta-analysis of the past 25 years of weight loss research using diet, exercise or diet plus exercise intervention', *International Journal of Obesity* (1997) 21, 941–947.

Negoianu, D. and Goldfarb, S. (2008) 'Just add water', *Journal of the American Society of Nephrology*, 19 (6), 1041–1043.

NHS (2013) 'Eat less saturated fat'. www.nhs.uk/Livewell/Goodfood/Pages/Eat-less-saturated-fat.aspx

Noakes, M., Keogh, J.B., Foster, P.R. and Clifton, P.M. (2005) 'Effect of an energy-restricted, high-protein, low-fat diet relative to a conventional high-carbohydrate, low-fat diet on weight loss, body composition, nutritional status, and markers of cardiovascular health in obese women', *American Journal of Clinical Nutrition*, 81 (6), 1298–1306.

Ottley, C. (2000) 'Food and mood', *Nursing Standard*, 15 (2), 46–52.

Parra, D., Ramel, A., Bandarra, N., Kiely, M., Alfredo Martinez, J. and Thorsdottir, I. (2008) 'A diet rich in long chain Omega 3 fatty acids modulates satiety in overweight and obese volunteers during weight loss', *Appetite*, 51 (3), 676–680.

Parker, B., Noakes, M., Luscombe, N. and Clifton, P. (2002) 'Effect of a high-protein, high–monounsaturated fat weight loss diet on glycemic control and lipid levels in type 2 diabetes', *Diabetes Care*, 25 (3), 425–430.

Peer, M. (2008) *You can be thin*. Sphere, London, UK.

Reddy, S.T., Wang, C.Y., Sakhaee, Y., Brinkley, L. and Pak, C.Y.C (2002) 'Effect of low-carbohydrate high-protein diets on acid-base balance, stone-forming propensity, and calcium metabolism', *American Journal of Kidney Diseases*, 40 (2), 265–274.

Samaha F.F., Iqbal, N., Seshadri, P., Chicano, K.L., Daily, D.A., McGrory, J., Williams, T., Williams, M., Gracely, E.J. and Stern, L. (2003) 'A low-carbohydrate as compared with a low fat diet in sever obesity', *New England Journal of Medicine*, 348 (21), 2074–2081.

Scientific Advisory Committee on Nutrition (2011) 'Dietary reference values for energy', www.sacn.gov.uk/pdfs/sacn_dietary_reference_values_for_energy.pdf, accessed 25/10/13.

Siri-Tarino, P.W., Sun, Q., Hu, F.B. and Krauss R.M. (2010) 'Meta-analysis of prospective cohort studies evaluating the association of saturated fat with cardiovascular disease', *American Journal of Clinical Nutrition*, 91, 535–546.

Skov A.R., Toubro S., Rønn B., Holm L. Astrup A. (1999) 'Randomized trial on protein vs carbohydrate in ad libitum fat reduced diet for the treatment of obesity', *International Journal of Obesity and Related Metabolic Disorders: Journal of the International Association for the Study of Obesity*, 23(5), 528–536.

Sreekumaran Nair, K. (2005) 'Aging muscle', *American Journal of Clinical Nutrition*, 81 (5), 953–963.

Stookey, J.D., Constant, F., Popkin, B.M. and Gardner, C.D. (2008) 'Drinking water is associated with weight loss in overweight dieting women independent of diet and activity', *Obesity*, 16, 2481–2488.

Taubes, G. (2008) *Good calories, bad calories: fats, carbs and the controversial science of diet and health*. Anchor, USA.

USDA Center for Nutrition Policy and Promotion (1998) 'Is total fat consumption really decreasing?' *Nutrition Insights*.

Van Ittersum, K. and Wansink, B. (2012) 'Plate size and color suggestibility: The Delboeuf illusion's bias on serving and eating behaviour', *Journal of Consumer Research*, 39(2), 215–228

US Department for Agriculture (2013) www.choosemyplate.gov, accessed 27/10/13.

Wansink, B. and Payne, C.R. (2008). 'Eating behaviour and obesity at Chinese buffets', *Obesity*, 16(8), 1957–1960.

Werle, C.O.C., Wansink, B. and Payne, C.R. (2011) 'Just thinking about exercise makes me serve more food: physical activity and calorie compensation', *Appetite*, 56 (2), 332–335.

Yancy, W.S. Jr., Olsen, M.K., Guyton, J.R., Bakst, R.P. and Westman, E.C. (2004) 'A low-carbohydrate, ketogenic diet versus a low-fat diet to treat obesity and hyperlipidemia: a randomized, controlled trial', *Annals of Internal Medicine*, 140 (10), 769–777.

CHAPTER 6

ACSM (2009) ACSM position statement on physical activity and weight loss www.acsm.org/about-acsm/media-room/acsm-in-the-news/2011/08/01/acsm-position-stand-on-physical-activity-and-weight-loss-now-available, accessed 05/08/13.

Andersen, R.E., Wadden, T.A., Bartlett, S.J., Zemel, B., Verde, T.J. and Franckowiak, S.C. (1999) 'Effects of lifestyle activity vs structured aerobic exercise in obese women: a randomized trial', *Journal of the American Medical Association*, 28 (4), 335–340

Anderson, O. (2013) 'Fat burning: train your metabolism to use up those calories', *Peak Performance*, www.pponline.co.uk/encyc/fat-burning-train-your-metabolism-to-use-up-those-calories-274, accessed 12/07/13.

Baker, C.W. and Brownell, K.D. (2000) 'Physical activity and maintenance of weight loss: physiological and psychological mechanisms', in Bouchard, C. *Physical Activity and Obesity*. Human Kinetics, Illinois.

BBC News, (18th October, 2013), 'Housework "not strenuous enough" for exercise targets'. www.bbc.co.uk/news/health-24570276, accessed October 18th, 2013.

Boutcher, S.H. (2011) 'High-intensity intermittent exercise and fat loss', *Journal of Obesity*, www.hindawi.com/journals/jobes/2011/868305/, accessed 01/10/13.

Burdette, H.L. and Whitaker, R.C. (2005) 'Resurrecting free play in young children: looking beyond fitness and fatness to attention, affiliation, and affect', *Archives of Pediatrics and Adolescent Medicine*, 159 (1), 46–50

Cooper Institute (2011) 'About us: working for the best preventative medicine solutions well into the future'. www.cooperinstitute.org/about, accessed 01/07/13.

Department of Health (11th July, 2011) 'UK physical activity guidelines. www.gov.uk/government/publications/uk-physical-activity-guidelines, accessed 23/10/13.

Durstine, J.L., Moore, G.E., Painter, P.L. and Roberts, S.O. (2009) 'ACSM's exercise management for persons with chronic diseases and disabilities', *Human Kinetics*, Illinois.

Epstein, L.H., Wing, R.R., Koeske, R. and Valoski, A. (1985) 'A comparison of lifestyle exercise, aerobic exercise, and calisthenics on weight loss in obese children', *Behaviour Therapy*, 16 (4), 345–356

Epstein, L.H., Wing, R.R., Penner, B.C. and Kress, M.J. (1985) 'Effect of diet and controlled exercise on weight loss in obese children', *The Journal of Pediatrics*, 107 (3), 358-361.

Garrow, J.S. and Summerbell, C.D. (1995) 'Meta-analysis: effect of exercise, with or without

dieting, on the body composition of overweight subjects', *European Journal of Clinical Nutrition*, 49 (1), 1–10.

Hagerman, F.C., Walsh, S.J., Staron, R.S., Hikida, R.S., Gilders, R.M., Murray, T.F., Toma, K. and Ragg, K.E. (2000) 'Effects of high-intensity resistance training on untrained older men. I. strength, cardiovascular, and metabolic responses', *The Journals of Gerontology*, 55 (7), 336–346.

Hunter, G.R., Byrne, N.M., Sirikul, B., Fernandez, J.R., Zuckerman, P.A., Darnell, B.E. and Gower, B.A. (2012) 'Resistance training conserves fat-free mass and resting energy expenditure following weight loss', *Obesity*, 16 (5), 1045–1051.

Jakicic, J.M., Wing, R.R., Butler, B.A. and Robertson, R.J. (1995) 'Prescribing exercise in multiple short bouts versus one continuous bout', *International Journal of Obesity Related Metabolic Disorders*, 19, 893–901.

Kane, A. (2013) 'How fat affects arthritis', Arthritis Foundation, www.arthritistoday.org/about-arthritis/arthritis-and-your-health/obesity/fat-and-arthritis.php, accessed 05/08/13.

Macrae, F. (January, 2008) 'Could simply standing up be as good for you as a workout at the gym?' Mail Online, www.dailymail.co.uk/health/article-505305/Could-simply-standing-good-workout-gym.html, accessed 03/09/13.

Martins, C., Morgan, L. and Truby, H. (2008) 'A review of the effects of exercise on appetite regulation: an obesity perspective', *International Journal of Obesity*, 32, 1337–1347.

Miller, W.C., Koceja, D.M. and Hamilton, E.J. (1997) 'A meta-analysis of the past 25 years of weight loss research using diet, exercise or diet plus exercise intervention', *International Journal of Obesity* (1997) 21, 941–947.

Pollock, M.L., Gaesser, G.A., Butcher, J.D., Despres, J-P., Dishman, R.K., Franklin, B.A. and Garber, B.E. (2011) 'ACSM position stand: the recommended quantity and quality of exercise for developing and maintaining cardiorespiratory and muscular fitness, and flexibility in healthy adults'. *Medicine and Science in Sports and Exercise*, 30 (6), 975–991.

Ross, R., Dagnone, D., Jones, P.J.H., Smith, H., Paddags, A., Hudson, R. and Janssen, I. (2000) 'Reduction in obesity and related comorbid conditions after diet-induced weight loss or exercise-induced weight loss in men: a randomized, controlled trial', *Annals of Internal Medicine*, 133 (2), 92–103.

Schuenke, M.D. and Mikat, R.P. (2002) 'Effect of an acute period of resistance exercise on excess post-exercise oxygen consumption: implications for body mass management', *European Journal of Applied Physiology*, 86, 411–417.

Swain, D.P., Abernathy, K.S., Smith, C.S., Lee, S.J. and Bunn, S.A. (1994) 'Target heart rates for the development of cardiorespiratory fitness', *Medicine and Science in Sport and Exercise*, 26 (1), 112–116.

Verger, P., Lanteaume, M.T. and Louis-Sylvestre, J. (1992) 'Human intake and choice of foods at intervals after exercise', *Appetite*, 18 (2), 93–99.

CHAPTER 7

ACSM (2009) see Chapter 6 references.

Bagnardi, V. Blangiardo, M., La Vecchia, C. and Corrao, G. (2001) 'Alcohol consumption and the risk of cancer: a meta-analysis', National Institute on Alcohol Abuse and Alcoholism. pubs.niaaa.nih.gov/publications/arh25-4/263-270.htm, accessed 22/08/13.

Biddle, S.J.H., Fox, K.R. and Boutcher, S.H. (2001) *Physical activity and psychological well-being*. Routledge, New York.

Boniface, S. and Shelton, N. (26th February, 2013) 'How is alcohol consumption affected if we account for under-reporting? A hypothetical scenario', *European Journal of Public Health*, doi: 10.1093/eurpub/ckt016.

Born, J.M., Lemmens, S.G.T., Rutters, F., Nieuwenhuizen, A.G., Formisano, E., Gerbel, R. and Westerterp-Plantenga, M.S. (2010) 'Acute stress and food-related reward activation in the brain during food choice during eating in the absence of hunger', *International Journal of Obesity*, 34, 172–181.

Department of Health (2013) Smokefree, smokefree.nhs.uk/ways-to-quit/, accessed 10/07/13.

Duncan, B.B., Chambles, L.E., Schmidt, M.I., Folsom, A.R., Szklo, M., Crouse, J.R. and Carpenter, M.A. (1995) 'Association of the waist-to-hip ratio is different with wine than with beer or hard liquor consumption', *American Journal of Epidemiology*, 142 (10), 1034–1038.

Epel, E.S. (2009) 'Psychological and metabolic stress: A recipe for accelerated cellular aging?' *Hormones*, 8 (1), 7–22.

Epel, E., Lapidus, R., McEwen, B. and Brownell, K. (2001) 'Stress may add bite to appetite in women: a laboratory study of stress-induced cortisol and eating behaviour', *Psychoneuroendocrinology*, 26 (1), 27–49.

Farley, A.C., Hajek, P., Lycett, D. and Aveyard, P. (2012) 'Interventions for preventing weight gain after smoking cessation', *The Cochrane Library*, onlinelibrary.wiley.com/doi/10.1002/14651858.CD006219.pub3/abstract.

Green Gym, www.tcv.org.uk/greengym, accessed 12/09/13.

Harvey, A.G. and Payne, S. (2002) 'The management of unwanted pre-sleep thoughts in insomnia: distraction with imagery versus general distraction', *Behaviour Research and Therapy*, 40 (3), 267–277.

Health and Safety Executive (2012) 'Stress-related and psychological disorders in Great Britain'. www.hse.gov.uk/statistics/causdis/stress/, accessed 27/07/13.

Kandiah, J., Yake, M., Jones, J. and Meyer, M. (2005) 'Stress influences appetite and comfort food preferences in college women', *Nutrition Research*, 26 (3), 118–123.

Maslach, C., Schaufell, W.B. and Leiter, M.P. (2001) 'Job burnout', *Annual Review of Psychology*, 52, 397–422.

Mineur, Y.S., Abizaid, A., Rao, Y., Salas, R., DiLeone, R.J., Gündisch, D., Diano, S., De Biasi, M., Horvath, T.L., Gao, X. and Picciotto, M.R. (2011) 'Nicotine decreases food intake through activation of POMC neurons', *Science*, 332 (6035), 1330–1332.

National Sleep Foundation (2013) 'How much sleep do we really need?' www.sleepfoundation.org/article/how-sleep-works/how-much-sleep-do-we-really-need, accessed 17/08/13.

Oliver, G. and Wardle, J. (1999) 'Perceived effects of stress on food choice', *Physiology and Behaviour*, 66 (3), 511–515.

Oxford Dictionary (2013) Definitions of stress in English. oxforddictionaries.com/definition/english/stress, accessed 27/07/13.

Paluska, S.A. and Schwenk, T.L. (2000) 'Physical activity and mental health, current concepts', *Sports Medicine*, 29 (3), 167–180.

Park, D.H., Yu, J. and Ryu, S.H. (2006) 'Alcohol and sleep', *Sleep, medicine and psycholphysiology*, 13 (1), 5–10.

Parsons, A., Ingram, J., Inglis, J., Aveyard, P., Johnstone, E., Brown, K., Frankiln, M. and Bermudez, I. (2009) 'A proof of concept randomised placebo controlled factorial trial to examine the efficacy of St John's wort for smoking cessation and chromium to prevent weight gain on smoking cessation', *Drug and Alcohol Dependence*, 102 (1-3), 116–122.

Patel, S.R and Hu, F.B. (2012) 'Duration and weight gain: a systematic review', *Obesity*, 16 (3), 643–653.

Rimm, E.B., Williams, P., Fosher, K., Criqui, M. and Stampfer, M.J. (1999) 'Moderate alcohol intake and lower risk of coronary heart disease: meta-analysis of effects on lipids and haemostatic factors', *British Medical Journal*, 7224, 1523–1528.

Snadlund, E.S. and Norlander, T. (2000) 'The effects of Tai Chi Chuan relaxation and exercise on stress-response and well-being: an overview of research', *International Journal of Stress Management*, 7 (2), 139–149.

Thompson Coon, J., Boddy, K., Stein, K., Whear, R., Barton, J. and Depledge, M.H. (2011) 'Does participating in physical activity in outdoor natural environments have a greater effect on physical and mental wellbeing than physical activity indoors? A systematic review', *Environmental Science and Technology*, 45 (11), 4660–4665.

University of Exeter Medical School (2013) 'Interdisciplinary research: Blue Gym', www.ecehh.org/research/#.blue-gym, accessed 12/09/13.

US Department of Health and Human Services (1994) 'Alcohol and hormones'. www.ncjrs.gov/App/Publications/abstract.aspx?ID=157975, accessed 01/07/13.

Van Dongen, H.P.A., Rogers, N.L. and Dinges, D.F. (2003) 'Sleep debt: theoretical and empirical issues', *Sleep and Biological Rhythms*, 1 (1), 5–13.

Wu, D. and Cederbaum, A.I. (2004) 'Alcohol, oxidative stress, and free radical damage', National Institute on Alcohol Abuse and Alcoholism. pubs.niaaa.nih.gov/publications/arh27-4/277-284.htm, accessed 01/07/13.

CHAPTER 8

Adams, S. (23rd August, 2012) 'NHS turning to weight-loss surgery to tackle obesity', *The Telegraph*, www.telegraph.co.uk/health/health-news/9494510/NHS-turning-to-weight-loss-surgery-to-tackle-obesity.html, accessed 15/07/13.

BOSPA (2013a) 'Is surgery the answer to your obesity problem?' www.bospa.org, accessed 02/09/13.

BOSPA (2013b) 'Gastric band'. www.bospa.org, accessed 10/08/13.

BOSPA (2013c) 'Gastric band post-op eating plan'. www.bospa.org, accessed 10/08/13.

British National Formulary, www.bnf.org.uk, accessed 02/09/13

Grilo, C.M. and Masheb, R.M. (2005) 'A randomized controlled comparison of guided self-help cognitive behavioural therapy and behavioural weight loss for binge eating disorder', *Behaviour Research and Therapy*, 43 (11), 1509–1525.

NHS Choices (2013) 'Weight loss surgery'. www.nhs.uk/Conditions/weight-loss-surgery/Pages/Introduction.aspx, accessed 02/09/13.

National Institute for Health and Clinical Excellence (2006) *Obesity: guidance on the prevention, identification, assessment and management of overweight and obesity in adults and children.* London.

Rapoport, L., Clark, M and Wardle, J. (2000) 'Evaluation of a modified cognitive-behavioural programme for weight management', *International Journal of Obesity*, 24 (12), 1726–1737.

US Food and Drug Administration (10th August, 2010) 'Meridia (sibutramine): market withdrawal due to risk of serious cardiovascular events'. www.fda.gov/safety/medwatch/safety information/safetyalertsforhumanmedicalproducts/ucm228830.htm, accessed 02/09/13.

INDEX